The Epidemiology of
Alzheimer's Disease
and Related Disorders

The Epidemiology of Alzheimer's Disease and Related Disorders

A.F. Jorm

National Health and Medical Research Council
Social Psychiatry Research Unit
Australian National University
Canberra, Australia

Chapman and Hall

London · New York · Tokyo · Melbourne · Madras

UK	Chapman and Hall, 11 New Fetter Lane, London EC4P 4EE
USA	Van Nostrand Reinhold, 115 Fifth Avenue, New York NY10003
JAPAN	Chapman and Hall Japan, Thomson Publishing Japan, Hirakawacho Nemoto Building, 7F, 1–7–11 Hirakawa-cho, Chiyoda-ku, Tokyo 102
AUSTRALIA	Chapman and Hall Australia, Thomas Nelson Australia, 480 La Trobe Street, PO Box 4725, Melbourne 3000
INDIA	Chapman and Hall India, R. Seshadri, 32 Second Main Road, CIT East, Madras 600 035

First edition 1990

© 1990 A.F. Jorm

Typeset in 10/12 pt Palatino by
Photoprint, Torquay, Devon
Printed in Great Britain by
St Edmundsbury Press Ltd, Bury St Edmunds, Suffolk

ISBN 0 412 31520 3

British Library Cataloguing in Publication Data

Jorm, A.F., *1951–*
  The epidemiology of Alzheimer's disease and related
  disorders.
  1. Man. Brain. Alzheimer's disease
  I. Title
  616.831
    ISBN 0–412–31520–3

Library of Congress Cataloging-in-Publication Data

Available

Contents

Preface

The aim in writing this book has been to give a scholarly integration of knowledge on the epidemiology of the major dementing disorders. Only one book has attempted this before – an edited volume by Mortimer and Schuman (1981). Because of the rapid growth of the field, their work is now out of date. Although it is still feasible for one person to read and integrate what is known about the epidemiology of major dementing disorders, this may soon be impossible; to write this book required that over 500 articles and chapters be read or re-read. The growth of knowledge is so rapid that, in a few years, the task would need to be broken up among several authors or simplified by only attempting a selective review.

Until recently, the epidemiological study of Alzheimer's disease and related disorders was largely confined to Britain and the Scandinavian countries, primarily because these countries have amongst the most aged populations in the world. More recently, the national base of the research has spread considerably. Other developed countries have rapidly ageing populations and are consequently investing more effort towards an understanding of the major dementing disorders. A notable trend has been the emergence of research on dementing disorders from countries outside Western Europe and North America. This is a very important trend, because epidemiological findings from Western Europe and North America may not be suitable for extrapolation to the rest of the world. Much of this new work is not well known because it is not available in English, but every effort has been made to review such work in this book.

This book was written on the suggestion of Tim Hardwick, formerly Senior Editor with Chapman and Hall, after he visited Canberra in 1987. After his departure from Chapman and Hall, editorial responsibility was taken by Christine Birdsall who was consistently helpful and encouraging. Several people provided specific help with aspects of the book: Helen Creasey and Henry Brodaty read an earlier draft and provided valuable suggestions for improvement; Trish Jacomb produced all the figures and did a number of literature searches; Penny Evans typed several drafts of the manuscript. Many of the ideas found in this book stemmed from articles previously published in journals, often with Scott Henderson or

Ailsa Korten as co-authors. I wish to acknowledge their significant contribution to these ideas and to thank them for many stimulating discussions on the epidemiology of dementia over the past five years.

Acknowledgements

Table 2.5 is reproduced from Berg (1988) with permission.

Figure 4.1 is reproduced from Jorm *et al.* (1987), with permission of Munksgaard International Publishers Ltd, Copenhagen.

Appendix A is reproduced from American Psychiatric Association (1987), with permission.

Appendix B is reproduced from McKhann *et al.* (1984) with permission of Dr E.M. Stadlan.

1 *Classification*

A prerequisite to the epidemiological study of dementing diseases is a method of classifying and assessing them. The study of these diseases can proceed using either very broad or quite specific classifications, depending on the purposes of the researcher.

Figure 1.1 shows a scheme for conceptualizing the classification of dementing diseases. The starting point in this scheme is cognitive impairment which is the major feature of these diseases. Cognitive impairment can be either congenital, as in mental retardation, or acquired during life. Our interest here is in acquired cognitive disorders. There are many types of acquired cognitive disorder, some of which generally involve an acute loss of cognitive skills (e.g. delirium, intoxication) and others of which are generally chronic conditions (e.g. dementia, amnestic syndrome). These syndromes can be further sub-divided into specific diseases, but Figure 1.1 shows this only for the dementing diseases, since they are the major focus here.

Ideally, epidemiological investigations should be carried out at the level of specific diseases, but this may sometimes be unnecessary. The

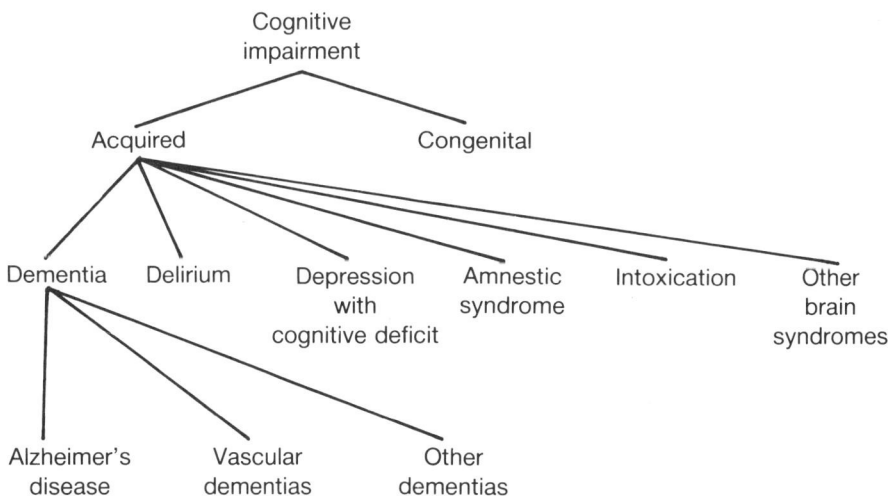

Figure 1.1 Scheme for classifying dementing diseases and related conditions.

level of specificity with which cognitive impairment is investigated by the epidemiologist depends on the purpose of the research. If, for example, the aim is to understand the aetiology of Alzheimer's disease, then nothing less than a diagnosis of Alzheimer's disease will be acceptable. However, other broader aims are possible. For example the researcher might be interested in the need for residential care beds for people with severe cognitive impairment. In this case, it may not matter whether the cognitive impairment is pre-existing or due to more recent cognitive decline, or what specific disease it is due to. To take another example, an epidemiologist might ask whether high education provides protection against cognitive decline in old age. Here, it is essential to distinguish cognitive decline from mental retardation, but not necessary to carry the process of differential diagnosis further.

Similar considerations apply in clinical practice. If the clinician has a specific treatment or prevention for a particular disease, then it is necessary for that disease to be diagnosed accurately. However, with the major dementing diseases, there are currently no specific treatments and the best available management may be possible with nothing more than a diagnosis of 'dementia'. It is for this reason that the syndrome of dementia exists at all. Dementia is not a disease state and might be expected to lose its usefulness as a category once effective treatment or prevention of specific dementing diseases becomes available. It may even turn out that what we today regard as specific dementing diseases are really just syndromes like dementia and that they will gradually lose their usefulness. The classification of diseases is always slowly changing, not necessarily toward some ultimate 'true' taxonomy, but towards a more useful system for guiding action in the areas of prevention, treatment and management.

The primary focus of this book is Alzheimer's disease and vascular dementia. These disorders are the most significant for epidemiological research because of the frequency of their occurrence and their social cost. However, many important epidemiological studies deal with cognitive impairment or dementia, rather than specific dementing diseases. These studies are also reviewed here because Alzheimer's disease and vascular dementia are believed to be the most important sources of cognitive impairment and dementia in the elderly.

1.1 CLASSIFICATION OF ALZHEIMER'S DISEASE

Alzheimer's disease was first described in 1906 as a progressive dementing disorder associated neuropathologically with senile plaques and neurofibrillary tangles. For much of this century it was classified as a pre-senile dementia and distinguished from the much more common senile dementia of the elderly. An important turning point was the report by Tomlinson *et al.* (1970) of their clinical and pathological study of demented elderly people. They found that most of these cases had the neuropathological hallmarks of Alzheimer's disease, while a smaller proportion had multiple infarcts. Following this report, the term **senile dementia of the Alzheimer type (SDAT)** became increasingly popular, but this was still commonly distinguished from presenile Alzheimer's disease. An influential editorial by Katzman (1976) took the final step in promoting a unitary concept of Alzheimer's disease by referring to both pre-senile and senile cases under the same rubric. Today, **Alzheimer's disease** is commonly used to refer to all cases irrespective of age of onset, but is sometimes reserved for neuropathologically confirmed cases, with the term **dementia of the Alzheimer type** being used for those where the diagnosis has been on clinical grounds alone.

The distinction between early and late forms of Alzheimer's disease has not altogether disappeared. Roth (1986) and his Cambridge group have argued for a distinction between Type I and Type II Alzheimer's disease. Type I tends to be of late onset and Type II of early onset, but age of onset is an imperfect indicator of the distinction. The distinction is principally justified on neuropathological and neurochemical grounds, with Type II cases having more widespread distribution of plaques and tangles and more extensive neurochemical changes. Clinical differences have been less well described, but include greater language dysfunction in Type II. While these differences could indicate separate disease processes, other interpretations are possible. Alzheimer's disease could be unitary with a tendency towards a more rapid course in early-onset cases. Early-onset cases would be likely to die at a more advanced stage of the disease because of this rapid progression and their decreased chances of dying from other age-associated diseases. By this means, early-onset cases could show more extensive neuropathological and neurochemical changes (Jorm, 1985). Contemporary epidemiological work tends to treat Alzheimer's disease as a unitary disorder while noting any age-of-onset differences, and it is this approach which is adopted here.

1.2 CLASSIFICATION OF VASCULAR DEMENTIA

Vascular dementia has received far less research attention than Alzheimer's disease and a consensus on its classification has yet to emerge. Part of the problem is that vascular dementia does not have a single pathological definition, unlike Alzheimer's disease which was originally linked by Alzheimer to the presence of senile plaques and neurofibrillary tangles. Therefore, clinicians have tried to link the clinical presentation of patients to various hypothesized pathologies.

An early influential typology was proposed by Roth (Mayer-Gross *et al.* 1954, 1960) who distinguished **arteriosclerotic** and **senile** psychoses. This distinction was based on Roth's careful clinical observations and has had a continuing influence even though the term arteriosclerotic dementia is no longer used. Not only did Roth's ideas guide much of the early epidemiological research on dementia, but his observations were later systematized by Hachinski *et al.* (1975) in the form of the Ischemic Score (discussed later in this chapter). This score still forms the major basis by which researchers distinguish Alzheimer and vascular dementias on clinical grounds. Later, the neuropathological studies of Tomlinson *et al.* (1970) were influential in showing that infarction was the most common cause of dementia in the elderly after Alzheimer's disease. However, the publication which has probably most influenced thinking about vascular dementia was a review by Hachinski *et al.* (1974) in which they argued that vascular disease causes dementia through infarcts rather than through atherosclerosis. They proposed the term **multi-infarct dementia (MID)** to describe this form of dementia and their term is now widely used.

In the years following the publication of Hachinski *et al.* (1974), the term multi-infarct dementia was used to refer to all vascular dementias and was treated very much as a unitary disorder. However, the subsequent advent of computerized tomography (CT) and magnetic resonance imaging (MRI) scans had a profound impact by providing a direct window on cerebrovascular disease. These scans allowed observation of small lacunar infarcts whose presence could not have been detected from clinical observation. This led to a distinction between lacunar dementia and multi-infarct dementia due to large infarcts. However, there is some dispute about whether multiple lacunes necessarily cause dementia and, indeed, whether a lacunar dementia exists at all (Scheinberg, 1988).

A similar controversy in classification has occurred with Binswanger's disease, a vascular dementia associated with ischemic white matter changes. In 1987, Babikian and Ropper were able to summarize only 47 pathologically verified cases of this vascular dementia in the world's literature. However, brain scanning has revealed periventricular white-matter lesions which have been interpreted as signs of Binswanger's disease. Roman (1987) has proposed the term **senile dementia of the Binswanger type** to describe this radiologically diagnosed disease and claimed that, together with Alzheimer's disease, it accounts for most cases of dementia in old age. Furthermore, Roman suggested that senile dementia of the Binswanger type is probably identical with lacunar dementia, whereas others (e.g. Wade and Hachinski, 1987) have argued that it is a different syndrome. However, there is dispute about the radiological diagnosis of Binswanger's disease. Morris (1989) was able to do a pathological examination of regions identified as white matter lesions by MRI and found no evidence of ischemic damage. He attributed the MRI findings to an accumulation of water in certain white-matter regions.

Sulkava and Erkinjuntti (1987) have proposed yet another type of vascular dementia which is due to cardiac arrhythmias and hypotension leading to cerebral hypoperfusion. They believe that one incident of hypoperfusion may be enough to lead to a dementing disorder called **vascular dementia of the haemodynamic type**.

Perhaps the most challenging proposal to come out of recent work on the classification of dementing diseases is that Alzheimer's disease may have an important vascular component. In a pathological study, Brun and Englund (1986) observed white matter changes in a majority of Alzheimer cases which they interpreted as incomplete infarctions similar to what is seen in the transitional zone surrounding complete infarction. Such changes were rare in normal brains. Brun and Englund speculated that cardiovascular dysfunction could lead to recurrent hypotension and cerebral hypoperfusion. This proposal has some similarity to that of Sulkava and Erkinjuntti (1987) and challenges the convention of distinguishing Alzheimer's disease from vascular dementias.

These important recent debates on the classification of vascular dementia have had little impact on epidemiological research. For this reason, vascular dementia is treated here as a global category which probably encompasses several different disorders. Greater refinement in epidemiological work on the topic must await some consensus on classification.

1.3 DIAGNOSTIC CRITERIA FOR THE MAJOR DEMENTING DISEASES

Research on dementing diseases is greatly assisted by the use of standard diagnostic criteria. These help ensure that different investigators are studying the same disorder. Older epidemiological research in this area tended to use broad definitions taken from textbooks or even the researcher's idiosyncratic concept of the disorder in question. Later research relied upon standardized criteria intended for clinical use and recent years have seen the development of criteria specifically intended for research purposes. The historical trend has been towards more precise and demanding diagnostic criteria.

Accurate diagnosis of specific dementing diseases is difficult to achieve during the patient's life. Definitive diagnosis must wait neuropathological evidence at autopsy or, rarely, from biopsy. In practice, however, neuropathological evidence is difficult to obtain or comes too late, so that both clinicians and researchers must rely on a 'probable' clinical diagnosis. The diagnosis of the syndrome of dementia (rather than specific diseases) is much more straightforward since it is defined in terms of clinical features rather than neuropathology. Criteria for broader syndromes, like cognitive decline or cognitive impairment, have not been proposed, probably because of their limited clinical usefulness and the ease of working down the diagnostic hierarchy as far as the syndrome of dementia. In this section, therefore, diagnostic criteria proposed for dementia or specific dementing diseases are examined.

1.3.1 DSM criteria

Among the most important diagnostic criteria are those published by the American Psychiatric Association in their *Diagnostic and Statistical Manual of Mental Disorders*. This has undergone several major revisions, the most recent being in 1980 (DSM-III) and 1987 (DSM-III-R). DSM-III-R distinguishes between organic mental **syndromes** and **disorders**. Organic mental syndromes are clusters of symptoms which occur together and are given a purely descriptive label, while organic mental disorders imply that the aetiology is known or presumed. Figure 1.2 illustrates this scheme. There are several organic mental syndromes of which dementia is the most important in the present context. The organic mental disorders are similarly divided into a large number of specific conditions. The figure shows only those disorders involving dementia and links them to this syndrome. However, similar linkages could be made between other syndromes (e.g. delirium) and specific disorders.

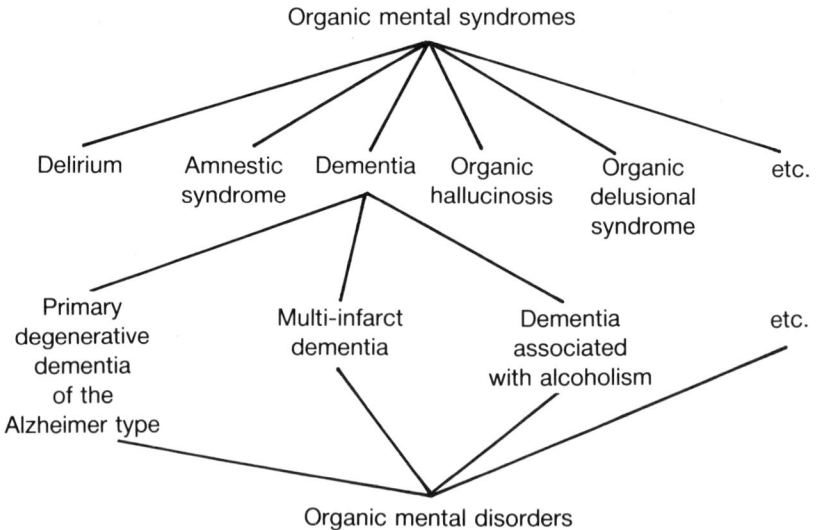

Figure 1.2   DSM-III-R taxonomy of organic mental disorders.

As well as proposing innovations in the taxonomy of organic mental disorders, DSM-III also specified the diagnostic criteria in much greater detail than had the earlier DSM systems. While this was an advance over earlier systems, the criteria were still lacking for epidemiological purposes. Jorm and Henderson (1985) discussed the problems in implementing the DSM-III criteria for dementia in this type of work. A major problem was that DSM-III treated dementia as a categorical state distinct from normal ageing. Thus, individuals had to be classified as either demented or non-demented. In the clinic the two may seem quite separate, but to the epidemiologist investigating the general population there will be a fine gradation in cognitive impairment. A judgement has to be made that a particular degree of cognitive impairment constitutes dementia rather than normal ageing. In practice, clinicians and researchers try to solve the problem by distinguishing gradations of dementia, using descriptions like mild, moderate or severe. Unfortunately, there was no systematic use of these terms because DSM-III did not define what degree of impairment constituted 'mild' and what 'moderate', etc. Henderson and Huppert (1984) have noted the huge variation in reported prevalence of mild dementia which reflects differing definitions of the term. The individual criteria for dementia also suffered from a problem of vagueness. Take, for example, the DSM-III dementia criterion: 'A loss of intellectual abilities of sufficient severity to interfere with social or occupational functioning.' Intellectual abilities are continuously distributed in the general population, so a decision had to be made as to how much loss is sufficient to satisfy the criterion. The assessment of 'loss' is also a problem. Strictly speaking, this requires measurement at two time points with a decline in scores between them. Very seldom are two measurements possible, so loss must be inferred, but DSM-III did not specify how. Liston and La Rue (1986) pointed out similar problems of vagueness with the criteria for multi-infarct dementia.

The new DSM-III-R criteria retain the basic taxonomic organization of the organic mental disorders developed for DSM-III, although there are some changes in nomenclature and additional categories to cover drug-induced mental disorders. The most important change in nomenclature for present purposes is the change from **primary degenerative dementia** to **primary degenerative dementia of the Alzheimer type**, with Alzheimer's name making its first appearance in the DSM system. More importantly, the diagnostic criteria for dementia were fully rewritten and overcame many of the particular problems raised with DSM-III. Appendix A shows the DSM-III-R criteria for dementia and specific dementing disorders. A most important feature is the recognition of the continuum from normal cognitive decline to severe dementia by the inclusion of criteria for the severity of dementia. Furthermore, the specification of each criterion is much more precise than for DSM-III and should result in greater agreement between diagnosticians. However, because these criteria are so new there are no data yet available on their reliability or validity.

1.3.2 ICD criteria

The International Classification of Diseases (ICD) system is intended to cover all diseases, unlike DSM which deals only with mental disorders. It was originally developed at the turn of the century for the coding of causes of death for statistical purposes. Its main purpose today is for keeping statistics on mortality and morbidity and indexing medical records. For epidemiological research on dementing diseases, probably the greatest importance of the ICD system is for the analysis of death certificate data.

The ICD is basically a listing of medical disorders without associated diagnostic criteria. However, in 1974 the World Health Organization published a glossary to go with the Mental Disorders section of ICD-8. This glossary gave basic descriptions of the characteristics of each disorder in an effort to ensure standardized usage of diagnostic terms.

When ICD-9 was introduced, a glossary was included as an integral part of the Mental Disorders section (World Health Organization, 1978). However, the descriptions in the glossary were quite rudimentary for the organic mental disorders. ICD-9 also involved some reorganization and relabelling of those disorders. In the USA there was dissatisfaction with ICD-9 which resulted in the development of a variant system, ICD-9-CM, for use in that country. This modification involved the inclusion of alternative diagnostic terms and new categories, and subsumed within it the DSM-III classification and terminology.

Although the ICD system has been used for epidemiological studies of dementia mortality, it has not provided diagnostic criteria of sufficient detail to be useful in clinic or field studies. However, the latest revision of the system, ICD-10, has made major advances in this respect. ICD-10 provides two sets of criteria: one for clinical use and one for research. The research criteria are much more detailed than those intended for clinical use. Table 1.1 shows the ICD-10 taxonomy of dementia disorders. An important feature of the research criteria for epidemiological use is that they recognize the continuous rather than categorical nature of these disorders by giving criteria for mild, moderate and severe levels of dementia. The criteria also describe in a fair degree of detail the types of information that need to be gathered to satisfy each criterion. Because the ICD-10 criteria have only recently been developed, no information is available on the reliability or validity of diagnoses made using them. However, given the detailed and specific nature of the criteria, we might expect a high degree of agreement between diagnosticians.

Table 1.1 ICD-10 taxonomy of dementia disorders (January 1989 draft)

F00	**Dementia in Alzheimer's disease**

F00.0 Dementia in Alzheimer's disease, presenile onset (Type 2)
F00.1 Dementia in Alzheimer's disease, senile onset (Type 1)
F00.2 Dementia in Alzheimer's disease, atypical or mixed type
F00.8 Other

F01   **Vascular dementia**

F01.0 Vascular dementia of acute onset
F01.1 Multi-infarct (predominantly cortical) vascular dementia
F01.2 Subcortical vascular dementia
F01.3 Mixed cortical and subcortical vascular dementia
F01.8 Other

F02   **Dementia in diseases classified elsewhere**

F02.0 Dementia in Pick's disease
F02.1 Dementia in Creutzfeldt-Jakob disease
F02.2 Dementia in Huntington's disease
F02.3 Dementia in Parkinson's disease
F02.4 Dementia in HIV infection
F02.8 Dementia in other diseases classified elsewhere

F03   **Dementia, unspecified**

DSM and ICD are the only systems which aim to provide criteria for all the major dementing diseases. However, there are a number of systems covering a more limited range of criteria which are of considerable importance to researchers.

1.3.3 NINCDS–ADRDA criteria for Alzheimer's disease

A Work Group on the Diagnosis of Alzheimer's Disease was set up in the USA by the National Institute of Neurological and Communicative Disorders and Stroke (NINCDS) and the Alzheimer's Disease and Related Disorders Association (ADRDA). The aim of the group was to establish clinical criteria for the diagnosis of Alzheimer's disease which could be used to select a homogeneous and relatively pure group of patients for research purposes. These criteria were published in a paper by McKhann *et al.* (1984) and are sometimes referred to as the 'McKhann criteria'. The group provided criteria for probable, possible and definite Alzheimer's disease. Since Alzheimer's disease can only be diagnosed definitely on the basis of neuropathological evidence, clinical evidence alone can only result in diagnoses of possible or probable Alzheimer's disease. These criteria are reproduced in Appendix B.

An important limitation of the NINCDS–ADRDA criteria is that they are intended for clinic-based research and would be difficult to implement in general population studies. Implementation of the criteria requires, for example, a history from an informant, a neurological examination of the sensory and motor systems, neuropsychological testing, a CT scan and blood tests, all of which are difficult to obtain in field survey conditions. Yet because of the potential inaccuracy of clinical diagnosis, anything less than this would be undesirable in research. This conflict between the need for diagnostic accuracy and the difficulty of obtaining the required information in field studies, has led Henderson and Jorm (1987) to question the feasibility of field studies of Alzheimer's disease using the latest diagnostic criteria. As the criteria have yet to be tried in such studies, the issue of feasibility remains unresolved.

The NINCDS–ADRDA criteria state that certain diagnosis is only possible with neuropathological evidence. Thus, the clinical criteria for probable Alzheimer's disease can be validated if neuropathological data become available later. There is evidence that the criteria can select cases with probable Alzheimer's disease with a reasonably high accuracy. Martin *et al.* (1987b) were able to carry out cortical biopsies on 11 cases clinically diagnosed with probable Alzheimer's disease. They found the diagnosis to be confirmed in every case. Tierney *et al.* (1988) have also carried out an autopsy study of 22 cases of probable Alzheimer's disease compared to 35 cases which were either normal or had other dementing disorders. The neuropathological diagnosis were carried out blind to the clinical diagnoses using several different criteria. Specificity of the clinical diagnoses was found to be high (89–91%), but sensitivity varied from 64 to 86% depending on the neuropathological criteria used. These results imply that the NINCDS–ADRDA criteria are useful for selecting out a group of patients who are likely to have Alzheimer's disease, but may exclude some true cases. Also worthy of mention is the study by Morris *et al.* (1988) of 26 cases who were clinically diagnosed using criteria which closely correspond to the NINCDS–ADRDA criteria. Many of these patients were only mildly demented at the time of diagnosis, but Alzheimer's disease was neuropathologically confirmed in all cases. The only study to report poor results with the NINCDS–ADRDA criteria is that by Boller *et al.* (1989). They found the sensitivity of Alzheimer's disease diagnoses to be high, but the specificity to be very low; in other words, the clinicians could accurately identify Alzheimer's disease when it was present, but tended to over-diagnose it in place of other dementing diseases.

1.3.4 Autopsy criteria for Alzheimer's disease

These criteria grew out of a conference held in the United States on the diagnosis of Alzheimer's disease in its earliest stages (Khachaturian, 1985). Participants were divided into a number of panels and the criteria were produced by the neuropathology panel. These autopsy criteria are the first attempt to standardize the neuropathological diagnosis of Alzheimer's disease and are unusual in that they propose diagnosis on neuropathological criteria alone, rather than in combination with clinical observations. It is usually held that certain diagnosis of Alzheimer's disease requires both clinical and neuropathological data.

The criteria specify the brain regions to be sampled and the number of plaques and tangles that must be observed in a microscopic field encompassing 1 mm^2 of the neocortex. The criteria specify plaque and tangle density using a sliding age scale such that a person under 50 years of age needs fewer of these changes to qualify as a case than, say, someone over 75 years. When a supporting clinical history is present, the criteria are allowed to be revised downwards to an unspecified degree. The sliding age scale is unusual and no justification for using it is provided. The implication is that what is normal in a very elderly person may constitute Alzheimer's disease in someone younger.

The validation of these neuropathological criteria is difficult to assess, but they can be usefully compared to clinician's diagnoses. Joachim *et al.* (1988) applied the neuropathological criteria to 150 cases diagnosed as having Alzheimer's disease which were contributed by over 100 physicians using their own clinical procedures. The cases ranged in age from 53 to 97 years. Despite the involvement of diverse physicians and the wide age range of the patients, there was 87% agreement between the clinical and neuropathological diagnoses.

1.4 CLASSIFICATION AND ASSESSMENT

The use of diagnostic criteria is only the first step in epidemiological research. In practice, the criteria have to be translated into a set of specific assessment procedures. Many standard assessment procedures exist for this purpose and these form the focus of the next chapter.

2 *Assessment*

Diagnostic criteria specify the various areas that should be assessed in the diagnostic process. However, they do not specify the particular questions to be asked of the subject or yield a quantitative score of some kind. When assessment is taken to this level of detail we have an assessment instrument. Instruments may assess dementing diseases at various levels of detail. At the most general level are those which assess global cognitive impairment and at the most specific level are instruments that yield diagnoses of particular dementing diseases. Where an assessment instrument yields a diagnosis, it could legitimately be described as a set of diagnostic criteria in its own right, with the critieria being stated in the most explicit detail possible. Thus, the distinction between diagnostic criteria and diagnostic instruments can be quite blurred.

There are a large number of assessment instruments available for dementia. These have been assembled, along with other geriatric assessment instruments, in a two-volume work by Israel *et al.* (1984). Those instruments which have been particularly useful in epidemiological studies are described below.

2.1 ASSESSMENT OF COGNITIVE IMPAIRMENT

Cognitive impairment can be assessed by numerous tests ranging from brief screening instruments to lengthy neuropsychological batteries. In epidemiological research it is the brief instruments which have proven most useful. The most basic use of such tests is as a stand-alone measure of global cognitive impairment. However, they can also be used in harness with diagnostic instruments, either as an integral component of the diagnostic process, as an initial screening test to select potential cases, or to assess severity in cases where dementia has already been diagnosed. There are numerous brief instruments available, the best-known of which are listed in Table 2.1. Although many cognitive impairment instruments have been used in epidemiological research, there are two which have been particularly influential: the Mini-Mental State Examination and the Information/Orientation scale. These are described in detail below.

Table 2.1 Brief instruments for assessing cognitive impairment

Test	Authors	No. of questions
Mental Status Questionnaire (MSQ)	Kahn *et al.* (1960)	10
Information-Memory-Concentration Test (IMC)	Blessed *et al.* (1968)	29
Abbreviated Mental Test Score (AMTS)	Hodkinson (1972)	10
Mini-Mental State Examination (MMSE)	Folstein *et al.* (1975)	11
Information/Orientation Test (I/O)	Pattie and Gilleard (1975)	12
Short Portable Mental Status Questionnaire (SPMSQ)	Pfeiffer (1975)	10
Cognitive Capacity Screening Examination (CCSE)	Jacobs *et al.* (1977)	30
Hasegawa Dementia Scale (HDS)	Hasegawa (1983)	11

2.1.1 Mini-Mental State Examination (MMSE)

The MMSE was introduced by Folstein *et al.* (1975) as a means for clinicians to grade the cognitive state of their patients. The MMSE consists of 11 questions which yield a score from 0 to 30 and takes only 5–10 minutes to administer. In field survey research, the MMSE has involved slightly modified items and scoring to that described by Folstein *et al.* for clinical use. The field survey version is shown in Table 2.2.

Although the MMSE yields a continuous score from 0 to 30, cutting points have been proposed for discriminating cases from non-cases. Folstein and McHugh (1978) proposed that scores of 24–30 be regarded as normal and 0–23 as indicating cognitive impairment. However, in American field surveys using the MMSE, two cutting points have been used: scores of 0–17 define cases of severe cognitive impairment and 18–23 cases of mild cognitive impairment.

A considerable amount of evidence has been collected on the reliability and validity of the MMSE. Folstein *et al.* (1975) examined test–retest reliability in a clinical sample over 24 hours and 28 days. The stability coefficient was high over both time periods (0.89 and 0.98 respectively). They also assessed reliability over 24 hours with different examiners and again found a high correlation (0.83). O'Connor *et al.* (1989a) found a test–retest correlation of 0.84 over eight weeks in a community sample, which is quite acceptable. Internal consistency reliability has been less impressive. In a large American community sample, Cronbach's alpha

Table 2.2   Mini-Mental State Examination as used in field surveys

Orientation: (10 points)
　　What is the year?
　　What is the season?
　　What is the date?
　　What is the day of the week?
　　What is the month?
　　Can you tell me where we are? (residence or street name required)
　　What city/town are we in?
　　What state are we in?
　　What county are we in? (What are the names of two streets nearby?)
　　What floor of the building are we on? (NOT ASKED IN COMMUNITY
　　　　SURVEY.)

Registration: (3 points)
　　I am going to name 3 objects. After I have said them, I want you to repeat
　　them.
　　Remember what they are because I am going to ask you to name them again
　　in a few minutes.

'Apple　　　Table　　　Penny'

Attention and calculation: (5 points)*
　　Can you subtract 7 from 100, then subtract 7 from the answer you get and
　　　　keep subtracting 7 until I tell you to stop? (Stop at 65.)
　　Now I am going to spell a word forwards and I want you to spell it backwards
　　　　(in reverse order). The word is WORLD. W O R L D.

Recall: (3 points)
　　Now what were the three objects I asked you to remember?

Language: (9 points)
　　What is this called?
　　　　(Show watch.)
　　What is this called?
　　　　(Show pencil.)
　　Now I would like you to repeat a phrase after me: 'No ifs ands or buts'.
　　Read the words on this page and then do what it says.
　　　　(Page says "CLOSE YOUR EYES.")
　　Take this paper in your right hand, fold the paper in half using both hands,
　　and put the paper down using your left hand. (3 points)
　　Pick the paper up and write a short sentence on it for me.
　　　　(Sentence must have subject and verb and make sense.)
　　Now copy the design that you see printed on the page.
　　　　(Design is interlocking pentagons. The result must have five-sided figures
　　　　with intersection forming a four-sided figure.)

* Subjects are given both these items and the item with the highest score is credited to
the total.

was 0.77 (Holzer *et al.*, 1984) and in an Australian community sample it was even lower at 0.68 (Kay *et al.*, 1985).

Validity of the MMSE has mainly been assessed using clinical diagnosis as the criterion. Folstein *et al.* (1975) examined validity by comparing demented, depressed and normal groups. The MMSE effectively separated these groups, with demented patients having the lowest scores, depressed patients with cognitive impairment the next lowest, followed by uncomplicated affective disorder patients and normals. In a further study of 137 consecutive hospital admissions, the MMSE was found to discriminate between dementia cases and all other diagnoses. Later, Anthony *et al.* (1982) assessed the validity of the MMSE in a group of 99 general hospital admissions, using diagnoses of dementia and delirium made by a psychiatrist as the criterion. Using the conventional 23/24 cut-point, they found it to be 87% sensitive and 82% specific in detecting dementia and delirium. Recent studies have also examined the MMSE's validity under field survey conditions. Kay *et al.* (1985) found it to be 100% sensitive and 82% specific against a diagnosis of moderate or severe dementia. While very encouraging, these results were somewhat circular in that MMSE items helped to make the diagnoses. A field survey by Folstein *et al.* (1985) did not suffer this limitation. They found 97% sensitivity and 56% specificity for dementia and delirium using the conventional cut-point. The lower 17/18 cut-point produced 63% sensitivity and 91% specificity. Similarly, O'Connor *et al.* (1989a) found sensitivity of 86% and specificity of 92% in their field survey using the conventional cut-point.

The MMSE has also been validated by correlating it with the Wechsler Adult Intelligence Scale. Folstein *et al.* (1975) found correlations of 0.78 with Verbal IQ and 0.66 with Performance IQ. Later, McHugh and Folstein (1979) reported a scatterplot of the relationship between MMSE and Performance IQ. This relationship is strong and linear up to IQ 100 and then levels off because of a ceiling effect in MMSE scores.

A recent study (Martin *et al.*, 1987b) was able to validate the MMSE against cortical biopsy results in a group of 11 Alzheimer disease patients. Plaque counts correlated −0.70 with the MMSE score, indicating that the test is a valid measure of disease severity.

Although the overall validity of the MMSE appears good, there have been questions raised about its suitability for the poorly educated. Anthony *et al.* (1982) were the first to draw attention to the potential limitations of the MMSE with this group. They found that it produced a higher rate of false positives amongst elderly people in the United States with less than nine years of education. O'Connor *et al.* (1989a), working in Britain, found that the MMSE had more false positives with elderly people who left school before 15, but more false negatives with the better educated. Field surveys using the MMSE have also found that it correlates with education (Holzer *et al.*, 1984; Escobar *et al.*, 1986;

O'Connor *et al.*, 1989b). While some researchers have regarded this correlation as clear evidence of biased items (e.g. Escobar *et al.*, 1986), others have concluded that it reflects true education-level differences in cognitive impairment (Jorm *et al.*, 1988a). This is a rather thorny issue which is discussed in greater detail in Chapter 7.

2.1.2 Information/Orientation (I/O) scale

Whereas the MMSE has had its greatest impact in the USA, the I/O scale has been mainly used in Britain. The scale was originally part of a brief assessment battery for the elderly known as the Clifton Assessment Schedule (Pattie and Gilleard, 1975). As well as the I/O scale, the Clifton Assessment Schedule had Mental Ability and Psychomotor Performance scales. The Clifton Assessment Schedule later had a Behaviour Rating Scale added in to it and became part of the Clifton Assessment Procedures for the Elderly (CAPE) (Pattie and Gilleard, 1979). However, of all these components, only the I/O scale has been influential in epidemiological work (Clarke *et al.*, 1986; Morgan *et al.*, 1987).

Table 2.3 shows the 12 items of the I/O scale. The content is similar to the earlier items of the MMSE, but the I/O scale is more limited in the scope of its items. However, the brevity of the scale and its acceptability to the public make it attractive for field surveys.

The validity of the I/O scale has mainly been studied in psychiatric hospital settings. Pattie and Gilleard (1975) assessed the scale with 100 consecutive admissions, using psychiatric diagnosis as the criterion. They found that a cutting point of 7/8 separated dementia cases from functional psychiatric disorders with 91% sensitivity and 93% specificity. A later cross-validation study (Pattie and Gilleard, 1978) replicated these

Table 2.3 Items of the I/O scale of the Clifton Assessment Schedule (Pattie and Gilleard, 1975)

1.	What is your name/full name?
2.	How old are you?
3.	What is your date of birth?
4.	What is this place/Where are you now?
5.	What is the name of this hospital/What is the address of this place?
6.	What is the name of this town/city?
7.	Who is the Prime Minister?
8.	Who is the President of the USA?
9.	What are the colours of the national flag/Union Jack?
10.	What day is it?
11.	What month is it?
12.	What year is it?

results, with 93% sensitivity and 90% specificity. The I/O scale has also been found to discriminate well between patients who are discharged within three months and those who stay longer, between patients requiring special psychogeriatric care and patients requiring ordinary care, and between patients who died within two years of admission and those who survived (Pattie and Gilleard, 1975, 1976). McPherson *et al.* (1985) examined the ability of the I/O scale to discriminate between various community-dwelling and institutionalized patients. They found that the scale discriminated dementing day-patients from in-patients and both these groups from various non-demented patients. Of most relevance for epidemiological purposes is the validity of the scale when used in field surveys. This has been evaluated by Morgan *et al.* (1987) who used diagnoses by psychogeriatricians as the criterion. They found a kappa coefficient of 0.83 between the I/O classification and the clinician's assessment of dementia. This corresponded to an overall agreement of 92%.

Less information is available about the reliability of the I/O scale. In their community sample, Morgan *et al.* (1987) reported an alpha of 0.84 which indicates acceptable internal consistency. Test–retest reliability has been reported for the CAS as a whole and is quite high over one and two years, but not for the I/O scale separately (Pattie, 1981).

2.2 DIAGNOSTIC INSTRUMENTS

If there is to be any cumulation of knowledge, it is necessary for epidemiological studies to be directly comparable to one another in terms of the diagnostic entities being researched. Standard diagnostic criteria attempt to achieve this, but still allow sufficient latitude for various researchers to interpret them slightly differently. The best way to ensure comparability is to use diagnostic instruments which involve a standard set of items and have an algorithm to arrive at a consistent diagnosis from these items. The diagnostic instrument then becomes a highly precise set of diagnostic criteria in its own right. The specific nature of diagnostic instruments has its price, however. When a particular set of items must be used, the criteria lose their cross-cultural transportability. For instance, a diagnostic instrument developed in Britain is unlikely to be usable without at least some modification in other English-speaking countries. When countries with other languages or very different cultures are involved, substantial changes might be necessary. It is for this reason that diagnostic criteria must be stated in reasonably general terms. Despite the problem of transportability, diagnostic instruments are of great importance to epidemiological research on dementia and several have been developed in recent years. These are described below.

2.2.1 Geriatric Mental State (GMS)

The GMS was developed by Copeland *et al.* (1976) and arose out of earlier standardized psychiatric interviews meant for younger adults. Two of these interviews, the Present State Examination (PSE) and Present Status Schedule (PSS), provided many of the items for the GMS. As well, other items were added specifically to suit the elderly, such as items to assess cognitive dysfunction and for rating comatose and delirious patients. The resulting interview takes an average of 30–40 minutes to administer. The GMS has been translated into several languages, including French, Spanish, German, Dutch and Danish.

As originally developed, the GMS standardized the information gathered from the subject, but the diagnosis was left to the clinician. Later, a computerized diagnostic algorithm called AGECAT was developed to standardize the diagnostic process as well (Copeland *et al.*, 1986). As it has been used to date, AGECAT only produces diagnoses of the dementia syndrome, rather than specific dementing diseases. To achieve specific diagnoses requires more information than the mental state data gathered by GMS. Nevertheless, GMS is particularly valuable for field surveys because it can be administered by a trained lay interviewer and AGECAT can be used to arrive at a clinical diagnosis. This obviates the need to employ experienced clinicians for this type of work. The disadvantage of AGECAT, however, is that it cannot yield immediate diagnoses because data must be entered into a computer.

The original GMS has spawned a number of variants as shown in Figure 2.1. In the United States, a longer interview, the CARE, was developed using many of the same items as the GMS. The CARE is described in greater detail below. As well, versions of the GMS suitable for use in community surveys were developed. The first of these, the

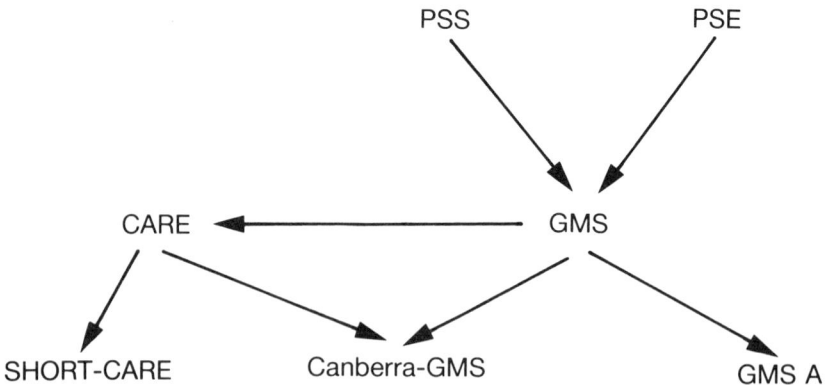

Figure 2.1 Historical connections among standardized psychiatric interviews.

Canberra-GMS, was developed in Australia using items from both the original GMS and the CARE (Henderson *et al.*, 1983). Later, algorithms were developed to allow the Canberra-GMS to arrive at DSM-III diagnoses of dementia and depression when used in harness with the Mini-Mental State Examination (Kay *et al.*, 1985). The other community survey version, the GMS A, was developed in Britain from the full GMS (Copeland *et al.*, 1988). This version takes only 15–20 minutes to administer. As with the full GMS, the AGECAT algorithm can be applied to the GMS A to arrive at standard diagnoses.

Several studies have been carried out to assess the reliability of the GMS. Reliability can be assessed in a number of ways. If two interviewers rate the responses of the same patients, then any variability must be due to differences between raters, while if the same interviewers rate a patient on two occasions, then any variability is due to inconsistency in the raters or changes in clinical state. Reliability can also be assessed at the level of final diagnosis or at the level of the individual items used in the interview. In the early years of the GMS, before the AGECAT diagnostic algorithm was developed, reliability studies necessarily focused on the individual items. Copeland *et al.* (1976) examined item reliability for the GMS and Henderson *et al.* (1983) did the same for the Canberra-GMS. The results were similar in both studies: reliability was high when different interviewers were rating the same patients, but lower when the same patient was rated on different occasions. Both studies also found less agreement between raters for items involving behavioural ratings than for items recording answers to direct questions.

The validity of diagnostic instruments like the GMS is difficult to assess. Inevitably it is done by using a clinician's diagnosis as the criterion, but clinical diagnoses are themselves in need of validation. At best, this type of validation study tells us whether the diagnostic instrument produces results consistent with a clinician's judgement. Studies which have compared the GMS and AGECAT with clinicians' diagnoses have found substantial agreement, using both psychiatric hospital patients and community samples (Copeland *et al.*, 1986, 1988). However, agreement was less satisfactory for geriatric hospital patients, mainly because AGECAT bases its diagnoses totally on the mental state examination, whereas psychiatrists may take other factors into account (Copeland *et al.*, 1986). For example, psychiatrists might distinguish between age-related and disease-related cognitive impairment, but AGECAT makes no such distinction. Similarly, depression associated with physical illness could be discounted by a psychiatrist as 'justifiable', but AGECAT does not take physical illness into account. To overcome the limitations of reliance on a mental state examination, GMS has recently been extended to incorporate a History and Aetiology Schedule (HAS) which gathers information from an informant. Data from HAS potentially allow dementia cases to be classified as Alzheimer's, multi-infarct and other forms of dementia (Copeland *et al.*, 1988), but results of this approach have yet to be reported.

2.2.2 Comprehensive Assessment and Referral Evaluation (CARE)

The CARE takes it parentage from the GMS. Both instruments arose out of an international study comparing psychiatric disorders in the elderly in London and New York (Gurland *et al.*, 1983). Whereas the GMS was primarily developed by the British research team, the CARE was the work of the Americans. The CARE takes most of the psychiatric content of the GMS, but has as well items relating to medical and social problems (Gurland *et al.*, 1977a); it is therefore much longer than the GMS, with 1500 items which take an average of 1.5 hours to administer. The interview draws information from a number of sources: self-report of the subject, test performance, interviewer observations and interviewer judgements. However, it does not incorporate either a physical examination or informant reports. The interview can be administered by trained lay interviewers as well as clinicians, but takes about a month of training for someone with basic interviewing experience. The lengthy administration and training time for the CARE, limit the usefulness of this interview.

Fortunately, the CARE has recently been reduced to a number of shorter versions, including the CORE-CARE with 314 items and the SHORT-CARE with 143 items (Gurland *et al.*, 1984). The CORE-CARE was produced by psychometric analyses of the original 1500 CARE items and, like the parent instrument, covers the psychiatric, medical and social domains. The SHORT-CARE, by contrast, covers only three areas of impairment in the elderly: dementia, depression and disability. The SHORT-CARE is therefore of most relevance in the present context. This interview takes a little over half an hour to complete.

Diagnoses of dementia using the SHORT-CARE (or the longer versions) can be achieved in two ways. The first involves the use of diagnostic criteria for 'pervasive dementia' specifically developed for the CARE instruments (Gurland *et al.*, 1982). These criteria are more specific than, say, ICD-10 or DSM-III-R in that they often specify particular CARE items. However, the diagnostic process still must be carried out by the interviewer and is not so specific that it can be applied as a computerized algorithm. However, Kay *et al.* (1985) have modified the pervasive dementia criteria somewhat so that they can be computerized and have applied this algorithm successfully to the Canberra-GMS. Gurland *et al.* (1982) have reported data on the reliability and validity of diagnoses using the pervasive dementia criteria. When the criteria for pervasive dementia are applied by different interviewers, there is a high degree of agreement, whether the interviewers be psychiatrists or social scientists. There is also strong agreement with face-to-face diagnoses of dementia using ICD-9 criteria. In fact, the diagnosis of pervasive dementia may be more valid than face-to-face psychiatric diagnosis. Gurland *et al.* (1982) carried out a one-year follow-up study to confirm the initial diagnoses. A number of cases diagnosed as demented by psychiatrists were found to be normal at follow-up, but this did not occur for the diagnoses of pervasive dementia. Although the various CARE interviews appear to yield reliable and valid diagnoses of dementia, criteria for the diagnoses of specific dementing diseases have not been produced. It is unlikely that they could be for the CARE, given that it does not involve a history from an informant or a physical examination.

The second approach to diagnosis of dementia from the CARE involves the use of continuous 'indicator scales'. A number of such scales have been developed from the CARE, the most important for the diagnoses of dementia being the Dementia and Depression scales. These two scales are particularly useful in guiding the differential diagnosis of dementia and depression. Subjects with low scores on both scales are regarded as non-cases, while subjects with high scores on one or both scales are assigned to the category (dementia or depression) from which their symptoms predominate (Golden *et al.*, 1983). The scoring of the indicator scales and placing of cut-offs is very simple and could be done by hand or readily programmed. This approach showed a high degree of agreement with clinical diagnoses in the original study, but requires cross-validation on a new sample to assess it properly. The main limitation of diagnosis via the indicator scales is that it forces everybody to be normal, depressed or demented, and does not allow for the simultaneous presence of both depression and dementia. However, this is a limitation of all categorical diagnostic systems and is best resolved by a dimensional representation of symptom severity as given by the original indicator scales.

2.2.3 Cambridge Mental Disorders of the Elderly Examination (CAMDEX)

The CAMDEX (Roth *et al.*, 1986) is the newest of the standardized diagnostic instruments. It focuses primarily on dementia, but also covers alternative diagnoses from which dementia must be differentiated, including depression, delirium and paranoid states. The CAMDEX uses more information sources than either the GMS or CARE. As well as a mental state examination of the subject, there is a mini-neuropsychological battery (the CAMCOG), an interview with an informant, a brief physical examination, and provision for recording laboratory findings and current medication. The interview with the subject takes about one hour and the informant interview 20 minutes. Use of the CAMDEX to date has involved medically qualified personnel and it is doubtful that it could be administered in its entirety by lay interviewers, given the nature of some of the information collected.

Because of the range of information gathered by the CAMDEX, it can be used to make clinical diagnoses of specific dementing diseases. At present, the instrument does not have a computerized diagnostic algorithm, so diagnoses are made by the clinician using detailed criteria associated with CAMDEX. Diagnostic criteria are given for four categories of dementia: senile dementia of the Alzheimer type (SDAT), multi-infarct dementia (MID), mixed SDAT/MID, and dementia secondary to other causes; as well as for delirium and various non-organic disorders. Roth *et al.* (1988) have also specified the CAMDEX items which can be used to meet DSM-III-R and ICD-10 criteria. However, a skilled clinician is still needed to translate from the items to the published criteria. The application of the items to standard diagnostic criteria is too loose to permit a computerized diagnosis.

To aid the diagnostic process, three continuous diagnostic scales have been developed from the CAMDEX items. The first was intended to measure degree of SDAT, but proved to be a general scale of organicity. The second measures MID, and the third depression. Normal individuals have low scores on all scales. Both SDAT and MID cases are high on the Organicity scale, but MID cases are high on the MID scale while SDAT cases are low. Depressed cases score high on the Depression scale but low on Organicity and MID. These three scales are relatively independent of each other and have high internal-consistency reliability. It is planned to use these scales as a basis for computerized diagnosis in the future, along the lines of AGECAT.

One of the most useful components of the CAMDEX is its cognitive examination. The CAMCOG incorporates the widely-used MMSE, but includes many other items to make up for omissions in the MMSE. It covers additional areas of cognitive function and has more detailed coverage of crucial areas like memory. The CAMCOG has eight subscales covering orientation, language, memory, praxis, attention, abstract thinking, perception and calculation. Although these purport to measure different areas of neuropsychological function, factor analysis of the items revealed one general factor accounting for most of the variance. This means that the CAMCOG can be treated as a unidimensional measure of general cognitive ability. When all CAMCOG items are added together it yields scores from 0–106, with a cut-off of 79/80 giving good discrimination between cognitively impaired patients and normals. The sensitivity and specificity of the CAMCOG has been reported to be superior to the MMSE, but unfortunately the criterion diagnoses were contaminated by the clinician's knowledge of CAMCOG performance.

Nevertheless, an important advantage of the CAMCOG over shorter instruments like the MMSE is that it avoids the ceiling effect which occurs when most people score close to the maximum.

Data on the reliability of the CAMDEX have so far been reported only with clinical samples. When different interviewers rated the same patients, agreement was found to be high on individual items and on the final diagnosis of cases as normal or demented. However, diagnostic agreement was lower when dementia was subdivided into specific categories. This disagreement resulted largely because of problems in differentiating mixed SDAT/MID from SDAT and MID alone. No data on the validity of the CAMDEX diagnoses is presently available. Ultimately, these need to be correlated with neuropathological findings.

The CAMDEX was developed in Britain and the initial work supporting its usefulness involved the same clinicians who developed it. However, Hendrie *et al.* (1988), working in the United States, have replicated much of the original research on the CAMDEX, showing its potential usefulness in other countries.

2.3 AIDS TO DIAGNOSIS

While standardized diagnostic instruments like the GMS, CARE and CAMDEX aim to collect all the information necessary to achieve a diagnosis, there are other instruments which are designed to assist one aspect of the diagnostic process. Such instruments have been influential in two important areas: the differentiation of AD from vascular dementia on clinical grounds, and staging of the severity of dementia. The relevant instruments for these purposes are reviewed next.

2.3.1 Differentiation of Alzheimer and vascular dementias

The differential diagnosis of Alzheimer and vascular dementias presents particular difficulties. To achieve this adequately requires both clinical and pathological data, but in epidemiological research only clinical observations are usually possible. Early epidemiological research involving the differentiation of these two types of dementia was generally based on Roth's clinical descriptions of **senile** and **arteriosclerotic** dementias (Mayer-Gross *et al.*, 1960). Roth's descriptions were later used by Hachinski *et al.* (1975) to derive an Ischemic Score. As shown in Table 2.4, this Score is based on 13 features which are weighted 1 or 2, depending on their importance, to yield a total from 0 to 18. Scores of 7 or more are regarded as indicating vascular dementia, while 4 or below indicates an Alzheimer dementia. The Ischemic Score has had a major impact on epidemiological research and is currently the standard approach to the clinical differentiation of Alzheimer and vascular dementias.

Table 2.4   Ischemic Score of Hachinski *et al.* (1975)

Feature	Score
Abrupt onset	2
Stepwise deterioration	1
Fluctuating course	2
Nocturnal confusion	1
Relative preservation of personality	1
Depression	1
Somatic complaints	1
Emotional incontinence	1
History of hypertension	1
History of strokes	2
Evidence of associated atherosclerosis	1
Focal neurological symptoms	2
Focal neurological signs	2

However, despite its widespread popularity, serious questions have been raised about the reliability and validity of this scale.

Only one study has been done on the reliability of the Ischemic Score. Gustafson and Nilsson (1982) had two clinicians complete the scale independently on 57 early-onset dementia cases. They found a correlation of only 0.39 between the two scores, which indicates a disturbing lack of agreement. A likely reason for such substantial disagreement is the vagueness of the Ischemic Score items. Simple descriptions like 'stepwise deterioration' and 'fluctuating course' are open to a variety of interpretations. Indeed, Roth (1981) has commented on the need for greater specification of the meanings of the Ischemic Score items and has given expanded descriptions of each. There have also been some systematic attempts to improve the Ischemic Score in this respect. Small (1985) has produced a Revised Ischemic Score which gives expanded definitions of items and allows weighting of each feature according to its severity and the clinician's confidence in the data available. Although this revised scale is likely to improve inter-rater reliabilty, no research on the topic has been reported. Another attempt to improve the specification of the Ischemic Score is incorporated within the CAMDEX. The CAMDEX collects information to allow the Ischemic Score to be calculated, but involves particular questions to be asked of the subject or of an informant or to be rated by the interviewer. Again, no reliability data are available, but the CAMDEX Ischemic Score is likely to be more satisfactory than the original.

In addition to the reliability problem, serious questions have been raised about the validity of clinical differentiation of vascular and

Alzheimer dementias. Liston and La Rue (1983) have reviewed the relevant studies using pathological diagnosis as the criterion and concluded that the validity of the Ischemic Score has yet to be adequately demonstrated. They argue that although a low Ischemic Score rules out vascular dementia, a high score does not necessarily indicate that a dementia is of vascular origin. This is because a vascular dementia is unlikely to occur without producing the sorts of clinical changes measured by the Ischemic Score. However, a high Ischemic Score may occur because of vascular lesions which are aetiologically unrelated to the dementia, as in a case where Alzheimer's disease is incidentally accompanied by a stroke. Liston and La Rue argue that the main use of the Ischemic Score is to aid the clinical diagnoses of Alzheimer's disease by exclusion of competing alternatives. Although the Ischemic Score may be inadequate for the positive diagnosis of vascular dementia, it has often been used in this way in epidemiological research and will result in an overestimate of the frequency of this type of dementia.

2.3.2 Staging of dementia severity

Until recently, diagnostic criteria for dementia have treated the syndrome as categorical in nature, being either present or absent. To clinicians there may often appear to be a gulf between normal ageing and dementia, but epidemiologists working in the general community observe a gradation from normal ageing to severe dementia. This gradation necessitates the use of adjectives like 'mild', 'moderate' or 'severe' when describing dementia. Unfortunately, these adjectives are used inconsistently from one investigator to another. The problem is particularly acute for mild dementia, where varying definitions have led to prevalence estimates ranging from 2.0 to 52.7% (Henderson and Huppert, 1984). To overcome this problem it is necessary to give criteria for different levels of severity. Two attempts to do this are the Global Deterioration Scale of Reisberg *et al.* (1982) and the Clinical Dementia Rating of Hughes *et al.* (1982). Only the latter scale has had influence in epidemiological research and merits detailed discussion here.

The Clinical Dementia Rating (CDR) was first described by Hughes *et al.* (1982), but a slightly revised version was subsequently produced by this research team (Berg, 1988). The newer version is shown in Table 2.5. It can be seen that the CDR distinguishes five stages, ranging from *healthy* to *severe dementia*. To arrive at a stage, a rater must score each area of functioning (memory, orientation, etc.) as independently as possible. Memory is given primacy in determining the overall stage. If at least three other areas are given the same score as memory, then the memory score corresponds to the stage. However, if three or more of the other categories are scored consistently higher or lower, they can

Table 2.5 Clinical Dementia Rating (CDR) of Berg (1988)

Criteria	No dementia CDR 0	Questionable dementia CDR 0.5	Mild dementia CDR 1	Moderate dementia CDR 2	Severe dementia CDR 3
Memory	No memory loss or slight inconstant forgetfulness	Consistent slight forgetfulness; partial recollection of events; 'benign' forgetfulness	Moderate memory loss, more marked for recent events; defect interferes with everyday activities	Severe memory loss; only highly learned material retained; new material rapidly lost	Severe memory loss; only fragments remain
Orientation	Fully oriented	Fully oriented except for slight difficulty with time relationships	Moderate difficulty with time relationships; oriented for place at examination; may have geographical disorientation elsewhere	Severe difficulty with time relationships; usually disoriented in time, often to place	Oriented to person only
Judgement and problem solving	Solves everyday problems well; judgement good in relation to past performance	Slight impairment in solving problems, similarities, differences	Moderate difficulty in handling problems, similarities, differences; social judgement usually maintained	Severely impaired in handling problems, similarities, differences; social judgement usually impaired	Unable to make judgements or solve problems

Community affairs	Independent function at usual level in job, shopping, business and financial affairs, volunteer and social groups	Slight impairment in these activities	Unable to function independently at these activities though may still be engaged in some; appears normal to casual inspection	No pretence of independent function outside home Appears well enough to be taken to functions outside a family home	Appears too ill to be taken to functions outside a family home
Home and hobbies	Life at home, hobbies, intellectual interests well maintained	Life at home, hobbies, intellectual interests slightly impaired	Mild but definite impairment of function at home; more difficult chores abandoned; more complicated hobbies and interests abandoned	Only simple chores preserved; very restricted interests, poorly sustained	No significant function in home
Personal care	Fully capable of self care		Needs prompting	Requires assistance in dressing, hygiene, keeping of personal effects	Requires much help with personal care; frequent incontinence

Score only as decline from previous usual level due to cognitive loss, not impairment due to other factors.

overrule the memory score. The CDR leaves the clinician free as to how to derive the scores for the various areas of functioning. However, in the original study of the CDR, Hughes *et al.* (1982) derived the scores using information collected via a standardized structured interview – the Initial Subject Protocol. This interview involved some cognitive testing of the subject and a number of questions to an informant. It would therefore be necessary for other users of the CDR to collect equivalent information on which to base scores.

The reliability of the CDR has been studied by Hughes *et al.* (1982). In a pilot study they found inter-rater reliability to be high ($r = 0.89$). In their main study of subjects rated 'normal', 'questionable' or 'mild', they found disagreement between raters in less than 5% of cases. In a later reliability study, Burke *et al.* (1988) found 20% disagreement in assigning CDR levels when different clinicians viewed videotaped assessments of the same patients.

Hughes *et al.* (1982) have also presented data on the validity of the CDR. The scale correlated very highly with short dementia screening tests and with informant ratings of memory and daily living impairment. However, these correlations may be spurious indicators of validity because the same test results were used by the raters to score the CDR. More satisfactory indication of validity comes from longitudinal follow-up of subjects 6–9 months later. If the CDR is valid, then subjects should either stay at the same stage or progress to a more impaired stage, but not move back to a less impaired stage. Hughes *et al.* found that all healthy elderly remained healthy, while all mild cases either stayed the same or progressed. With questionable cases, most stayed the same, some progressed, but only one was rated healthy. This pattern of results supports the validity of the CDR. In a later study of the CDR, Berg *et al.* (1984) followed up subjects rated as mild. After one year, half progressed to moderate or severe dementia and half remained mild. Berg *et al.* examined psychometric, clinical, electrophysiological and radiological data in an effort to predict those cases which progressed. Although all subjects were supposed to be functioning at roughly the same level at entry to the study, certain psychometric tests were found to predict subsequent decline. In other words, there was some hetero-geneity within this group of mild dementia sufferers in terms of cognitive function, such that the more impaired were the ones who tended to progress.

Thus, in categorizing subjects into stages, there is some loss of information which would be available if a continuous score had been used. It is noteworthy that one of the predictors of subsequent decline was an aphasia battery. Roth *et al.* (1986) have criticized the CDR because it places too much weight on memory. Subjects may receive the same CDR stage even though some have aphasic difficulties and others not. The results of Berg *et al.* (1984) indicate that language function should be taken into account in any staging scheme.

Staging schemes are basically supplements to standard diagnostic criteria. Earlier diagnostic criteria were based on categorical notions of dementing diseases, but newer ones like DSM-III-R and ICD-10 incorporate some staging of severity. It is therefore likely that separate staging instruments will become less important for future epidemiological research.

2.4 GUIDES TO ASSESSMENT AND DIAGNOSIS

In recent years, consensus statements have been published in both Britain and the United States which provide general guidelines on assessment and diagnosis, but do not constitute either diagnostic criteria or assessment instruments in their own right. These publications are too recent to have had an impact on epidemiological research, but may do so in the future, so are worthy of discussion here.

In Britain, the Medical Research Council (1987) has published a booklet describing recommendations of data to be collected in studies of Alzheimer's disease. By encouraging the collection of similar information across studies, it was hoped that data from different projects could be more readily compared and pooled and that conflicting results could be more easily accounted for. The recommendations give the minimum clinical information required to allow the diagnosis of dementia, the grading of its severity and the clinical diagnosis of the cause of the dementia. They also specify the pathological information needed to diagnose Alzheimer's disease and vascular dementia. However, the recommendations do not pretend to be diagnostic criteria in their own right. Rather, they specify information which may be helpful in meeting standard criteria such as NINCDS–ADRDA. The recommendations fall into four areas:

1. basic demographic data about the subject;
2. history from an informant;
3. examination of the subject;
4. neuropathological assessment.

In the first three of these areas, the recommendations specify particular questions to be asked, most of which come from established instruments like the MMSE, GMS and CAMDEX. The neuropathological recommendations specify the clinical information to be collected, brain regions to be studied, the neuropathological investigation techniques to be used, and the alternative dementing diseases which have to be excluded. The MRC recommendations are not regarded as final and are to be revised in future years.

In the United States, the National Institutes of Health (1987) have produced a consensus statement on the differential diagnosis of dementing diseases. This statement was the work of a panel with representatives from various disciplines. The consensus statement covered five questions:

1. What is dementia?
2. What are the dementing diseases, and which of them can be readily arrested or reversed?
3. What should be included in the initial evaluation of dementia?
4. What diagnostic tests should be performed, and when are these tests indicated?
5. What are the priorities for future research on diagnosing the dementias?

The statements on evaluation and diagnostic tests are primarily aimed at practitioners, but will no doubt have some influence on research as well. They specify the types of information to be collected and summarize the strengths and weaknesses of various diagnostic tests.

Although neither the British or American recommendations have yet had time to influence epidemiological research, it is instructive to look at past research in light of these recommendations. It is unlikely that early studies would adequately meet these standards, limiting the weight which can be placed on their results.

3 *Epidemiological research methods*

This chapter describes epidemiological research methods which have been used in the study of dementing diseases. It prepares the way for later chapters where a basic knowledge of these methods is assumed. Although the research methods used to study dementing diseases are, in principle, no different from those used for other diseases, their application to dementia sometimes presents unusual difficulties. Such potential problems form an important theme of this chapter.

Epidemiology aims to study the distribution of diseases in a population. In the early stages of epidemiological enquiry about a disease, research will often focus simply on describing the frequency of its occurrence in a population and its effects on mortality. While of some relevance for public health efforts, this sort of descriptive epidemiology contributes little to an understanding of the disease. The latter purpose is best served by studies searching for differences in disease occurrence between populations. The populations compared may differ in sociodemographic characteristics (e.g. sex, age, race) or may be defined in terms of differential exposures to potential risk factors (e.g. diet, industrial chemicals). When a disease is poorly understood, epidemiological studies of this sort will tend to be exploratory, with a large number of potential associations investigated in the hope that something will turn up. Much epidemiological research on dementing diseases is at this stage. When a disease is better understood, research becomes more theory-driven and can test specific aetiological hypotheses. Eventually, understanding of a disease may reach the point where preventive efforts become possible, and epidemiological research can evaluate the effectiveness of these. We begin by examining the methodology of the more descriptive types of epidemiological research, which are concerned with estimating prevalence, incidence and mortality, and then proceed on to research methods for investigating risk factors.

3.1 PREVALENCE STUDIES

The **prevalence** of a disease is of the number of cases in a population at a particular time. If the prevalence is divided by the number of people at risk, then we have a **prevalence rate**. The prevalence rate is often simply abbreviated to prevalence, giving the latter term a dual meaning. In studies of dementing diseases, prevalence is generally estimated at a particular point in time, giving a **point prevalence**, but occasionally studies are carried out of prevalence during a particular period (e.g. six months or a year), giving a **period prevalence**.

3.1.1 Defining a case

The notion of prevalence is based on the assumption that a population can be neatly divided into cases and non-cases. This can sometimes present problems. For example, with infectious diseases there will be cases which are undetected due to non-invasive colonization or sub-clinical infection. However, with chronic diseases of ageing the problem is much greater because the features of the disease will often be present in normal aged individuals. One explanation for this shading of ageing into disease is that many aged people suffer from subclinical or pre-clinical disease (e.g. Broe, 1988). A more radical view is that diseases of ageing are continuous with normal ageing rather than distinct disease processes (e.g. Dixon, 1988; Storandt *et al.*, 1988). Either way, it is not easy to define the point at which a person moves from normal ageing to becoming a case of, say, Alzheimer's disease. The cut-off chosen will, of course, affect the prevalence of the disease. Thus, with some diseases there is no true prevalence rate, but a variety of equally valid rates dependent on the exact definition of the disease in question. This is a theme which is discussed in greater depth in Chapter 4.

3.1.2 Types of prevalence studies

A prevalence study must locate all the cases in a population. The ideal method of achieving this would be to examine every individual in the population. Sometimes this is possible, as when Essen-Möller *et al.* (1956) were able to arrange psychiatric examinations of virtually every inhabitant of a small rural district in southern Sweden. Generally, however, a population is too large, or the personnel resources available are too small, to allow this. There are basically two alternatives to a complete population study: (1) to develop a register of cases in contact with services, or (2) to examine a representative sample of the total population.

Case registers provide a relatively cheap means of case identification. However, their limitation is that they only cover cases in contact with services. For some of the rarer dementing diseases it may be reasonable to expect that all cases will come in contact with services (e.g. dementia due to AIDS). However, with the major dementing diseases, such as

Alzheimer's and vascular dementias, many cases may be missed. The effectiveness of a case register will also depend on the services used as a basis for detecting cases. At one extreme are case register studies based on specialist psychiatric services (e.g. Adelstein, 1968; Wing and Hailey, 1972) and, at the other, registers which involve general practitioners, district nurses and nursing homes (Nielsen, 1962; Åkesson, 1969). The latter type of study will inevitably detect more cases. In some situations, a case register might be a very sensitive method of case detection, as in Bremer's (1951) study of an isolated Norwegian fishing village. During the period of investigation, Bremer was the sole focus of health care and had an extensive knowledge of the small community, enabling him to record all cases of psychiatric disorder, including dementia. While case registers will generally result in an underestimation of case numbers, it is possible to cast a very broad net, resulting in some false positives. The solution here is to combine the case register method with personal examination of all potential cases. As an example, Åkesson (1969) used not only medical sources of potential cases, but also social agencies and key informants such as clergy. He found these latter sources of information to be the most useful. Åkesson personally examined all persons reported as possibly suffering from a dementing disease and found that many were not demented. Without the second-phase personal examination, the broad case-detection net would have led to an overestimation of prevalence.

When dealing with a large population, the alternative to the case register is a field survey of a representative sample. Since dementing diseases are most prevalent in the elderly, samples are often drawn exclusively from this age group. Because the very elderly are rare, but yield a large number of cases, they may be over-sampled relative to the younger elderly. An example of such a study is that of Campbell *et al.* (1983) in a New Zealand town. These researchers focused their study on people aged 65 or over. Subjects were sampled at random, but stratified by age. Thus, a 1 in 20 sample was taken of those aged 65–74, a 1 in 6 sample of 75–79-year-olds, and a complete sample of those 80+. The use of representative samples allows prevalence estimates to be made for quite large populations. For example, Sulkava *et al.* (1985a) studied the prevalence of severe dementia for the whole of Finland, sampling 8000 people from a total population of 4.8 million.

Although sampling schemes may reduce the work-load in carrying out prevalence studies, the task of doing a full diagnostic examination on each subject may still be labour intensive, given the comparatively small yield of cases. To overcome this problem, two-phase designs are often used in field surveys. This involves an initial screening survey of all subjects and then a more intensive investigation of possible cases. If the study is estimating the prevalence of specific dementing diseases as well as global dementia, a three-phase design may sometimes be necessary. For example, in a survey of a US urban population, Folstein *et al.* (1985) first used the MMSE to screen for cognitive impairment. In the second phase, psychiatrists did house interviews with subjects likely to be cases. Finally, all cases of dementia were brought into a clinic for diagnosis of the specific dementing disease. While efficient of personnel, multi-phase assessment may result in unacceptably high rates of subject loss. Thus, in Folstein *et al.*'s study there were response rates of 75, 67 and 78%, respectively, in the three phases. While each of these is reasonably good, the compounding effect gives only a 39% response $(0.75 \times 0.67 \times 0.78)$ over the three stages.

3.1.3 Uses of prevalence studies

Typically, prevalence studies deal with a single population. Such studies can be of practical value in determining service needs for that population, but are otherwise uninformative. Of somewhat greater interest is the comparison of prevalence across populations. Unfortunately, because prevalence rates are so influenced by the definition of what is a case, it is meaningless to compare prevalence rates across different studies unless identical definitions are used. However, within a given geographically-defined population, it is possible to compare subgroups, e.g. sex, age and socio-economic differences. This assumes, of course, that the sample size is large enough to allow rates to be estimated for subgroups. Because of sample size limitations, many early prevalence studies simply reported a crude rate for people aged 60+ or 65+, which is not overly useful. Rarely, the same case ascertainment procedures are used in different geographic locations, making direct comparisons of prevalence rates possible. A good example is the US–UK Cross-National Project (Copeland *et al.*, 1987a) which compared the prevalence of dementia in New York and London using the same standardized interview and diagnostic algorithm. Prevalence was found to be higher in New York than London. Although such differences between populations are of great interest to epidemiologists, they can arise in two ways. Either the two populations differ in number of cases arising or in the duration of survival of those cases. From a theoretical point of view, the greatest interest lies in differences in the number of cases arising. For such purposes we need studies of incidence rather than prevalence.

3.2 INCIDENCE STUDIES

Incidence refers to the number of new cases arising in a population over a period of time, usually one year. An **incidence rate** can be calculated by dividing the number of new cases by the size of the population at risk. Often the term incidence is used as a synonym for the incidence rate. Although the idea of an incidence rate is conceptually straight-forward, matters are confused by there being two ways of measuring it. These differ in the way the size of the population at risk is calculated. The simplest is the **cumulative incidence rate** which is calculated by dividing the number of new cases by the number of people initially at risk. Those who are free of the disease at the beginning of the period are regarded as the number at risk. The cumulative incidence rate is the one generally used in studies of dementia incidence. The second measure is the **person–time incidence rate** or **force of morbidity** in which the denominator is the person-years of observation. The basic difference between the two is that the former continues to include an individual in the denominator even if they develop the disease during the period of observation, while the latter only includes the disease-free time of each individual in the denominator.

3.2.1 Defining new cases

In discussing prevalence, it was noted that splitting a population into cases and non-cases can be difficult for dementing diseases. Estimating incidence is even harder because it requires that the onset of new cases be measured. For a rapidly progressing dementia, specifying a point of onset would be easier than for a slowly progressing one. For example, with a typical late-onset case of Alzheimer's disease, it requires a somewhat arbitrary cut-off for determining when a person moves from normal ageing to diseased ageing. In fact, rather than measure the onset of the disease, incidence studies typically measure entry to some stage of severity. Because mild dementia presents some difficulties of assess-ment, onsets are often defined in terms of moderate-to-severe dementia. Thus, a person who suffered from mild dementia at the beginning of an observation period, and progressed to moderate dementia during the period, would be defined as a new case even though there has not been a new onset of disease in any categorical sense. Admittedly, the concept of incidence can even have problems when applied to infectious diseases, but it becomes much more strained when applied to chronic diseases of ageing.

3.2.2 Types of incidence studies

Because incidence refers to the onset of new cases over a period of time, incidence studies are necessarily longitudinal. The population under study must be assessed at the beginning of the observation period and also at the end. If person–time incidence rate is being estimated, then the onset of new cases during the period has to be dated. In addition, because new cases are uncommon, incidence studies require quite large samples to arrive at stable incidence estimates. In view of these demanding requirements, it is understandable that incidence studies of dementing diseases are far less common than prevalence studies.

The methods of case ascertainment in incidence studies are basically the same as in prevalence studies. Researchers tend to use either case registers, which vary considerably in the breadth of their case detection net, or else carry out longitudinal field surveys. The period of observation for incidence studies varies considerably, ranging from one year to decades.

3.2.3 Uses of incidence studies

Incidence rates are useful for uncovering differences between populations in disease onsets and may lead to the discovery of aetiological factors. However, most incidence studies of dementing diseases are, unfortunately, fairly useless for this purpose. Because the sample sizes required to estimate incidence rates are so large, many studies report only crude incidence rates for people aged 60+ or 65+. Such crude incidence rates are not directly comparable from one study to another because of varying definitions of what is a case and of the point at which case onset occurs. Furthermore, for diseases where the incidence is heavily influenced by the proportion of the population who are very elderly, crude incidence rates may differ between populations because of varying age distributions. Thus, in an ageing community where the very elderly are a substantial proportion of the total elderly, incidence is likely to be higher than in a community where the very elderly are a less prominent component of the total elderly.

To provide useful aetiological clues, incidence studies need to provide comparisons between differing populations. These comparisons might involve sociodemographic variables like age, sex and race, or differences in exposures to potential risk factors. Where two populations are defined in terms of the presence or absence of some potential risk factor and incidence is compared for the two populations, we have a **cohort study**. Such studies are described in greater detail later in the chapter.

3.2.4 Lifetime risk

Closely related to incidence is the concept of lifetime risk. This gives the risk for developing a disorder between birth and a particular age. The upper age chosen is arbitrary, but can be regarded as the end of some hypothetical lifespan. The lifetime risk is really a cumulative incidence rate for a lifespan. In principle, it could be measured by following a group of individuals from birth until the age of interest. However, in practice, some individuals will die before they reach the target age without developing the disorder. For this reason, lifetime risk cannot be directly measured, but can be estimated if it is assumed that, had these individuals not died early, they would have had the same risk of developing the disease as those who did survive. If the individuals dying early would have had an increased risk of developing the disorder, had they lived, then this assumption is not met. An example would be if males are likely to die earlier than females, but have less risk of developing Alzheimer's disease. Lifetime risk estimates for Alzheimer's disease based on data from both sexes would then be overestimates.

Table 3.1 Hypothetical data on the incidence of dementia, demonstrating the calculation of lifetime risk

Age period	Cumulative incidence rate over period	Proportion without onset
0 – 54	0	1.00
55 – 59	0.01	0.99
60 – 64	0.03	0.97
65 – 69	0.05	0.95
70 – 74	0.10	0.90
75 – 79	0.15	0.85

Lifetime risk $= 1 - (1.00)(0.99)(0.97)(0.95)(0.90)(0.85) = 0.30$.

Lifetime risk can be estimated by the product-limit method. This method requires knowledge of age-specific incidence rates up to the age of interest. Table 3.1 shows a set of age-specific incidence rates which have been expressed as proportions. Next to these is the proportion of the sample surviving each age period without onset of the disease. This is simply 1 minus the incidence rate. The lifetime risk is then calculated by multiplying together these latter proportions and subtracting the resulting product from 1. In the example, the lifetime risk of developing the disease up to age 79 is 0.30, or 30%. Lifetime risk is of considerable theoretical interest, because some theories involve specific predictions about the upper limit of risk. For example, Chase *et al.* (1983) have pointed out that if Alzheimer's disease was transmitted by an autosomal dominant gene, then first-degree relatives of cases would have a maximum lifetime risk of around 50%. The rest of the population would have a maximum lifetime risk of considerably less than this, with the exact value depending on the frequency of the Alzheimer gene in the population.

3.3 STUDIES OF MORTALITY AND SURVIVAL

The effects of dementing diseases on deaths in a population has attracted much epidemiological research. Such research has addressed two separate questions. The first concerns the frequency of deaths due to dementing diseases in the total population, while the second focuses specifically on those with dementing diseases and asks how their survival is affected compared to non-demented controls.

3.3.1 Mortality rates

Mortality or **death rates** express the proportion of a population dying from a disease by dividing the number of deaths by the size of the population in question. Usually death rates are calculated over a period of a year. Although the conventional approach is to use the population size as the denominator, some researchers have divided the number of deaths from a dementing disease by the total of all deaths in the population (Aubert *et al.*, 1987). Neither approach can be regarded as superior to the other. They simply reflect differing emphases. One looks at deaths from a disease in the context of the living population, and the other in the context of the dying population.

The major problem in studying mortality rates from dementing diseases is establishing that one of these diseases was the cause of death. The standard source of data for such research is death certificate records which have been classified by the most recent version of the ICD criteria. Death certificate records are readily available in many countries. There is an International Standard Death Certificate which allows recording of the immediate cause of death, conditions giving rise to the immediate cause, and the underlying cause of death. Published statistics are generally based on the single underlying cause of death, but some countries (e.g. Norway, USA) analyse multiple causes for each death. While the death certificate system may work for many diseases, it has great difficulties with the dementing diseases. Although these diseases may have effects on mortality, they will not generally be the sole disease present at death and may not be regarded by the attending physician as a cause of death. Where death certificate data have been checked for people known to have a dementing disease, there has been found to be substantial under-reporting on death certificates (Martyn and Pippard, 1988). This situation is likely to be worse in countries where only the underlying cause of death appears in official statistics compared to countries where multiple causes are analysed. Despite these difficulties, death certificate data have attracted the interest of researchers because they are available for whole countries and are readily accessible. Such data have been used to study regional differences in deaths from dementing diseases (Vogt, 1986), historical trends in dementia mortality (Newman and Bland, 1987) and age differences (Chandra *et al.*, 1986a).

3.3.2 Survival in dementia cases

There has been considerable interest in whether dementing diseases affect survival. Survival can be measured in a number of ways. Perhaps the simplest is to measure the **mean duration** of survival. This is a theoretically important measure because it relates prevalence to incidence. The prevalence of a disease equals the incidence times the mean duration of survival. The other two measures used are the **cumulative survival rate** and **cumulative mortality rate**. These are the converse of each other. The cumulative survival rate is the proportion of cases alive at the beginning of a time interval who are still alive at the end of the interval. The cumulative mortality rate is 1 minus the cumulative survival rate. Typically, survival is studied over a period of years and calculated on a yearly basis until there are no survivors.

Although the study of survival is, in principle, quite simple, the application to dementing diseases can present problems. Survival must be studied from some meaningful point in time. The most meaningful choice is the date of disease onset, but it is impossible to determine the onset of pathology for dementing diseases (or any other diseases for that matter). In practice, onset can be defined as the point at which clinically significant changes occur, e.g. impairment of activities of daily living. With dementing diseases, particularly slowly progressing ones, formal recognition of the disease may come quite some time after such changes. The dating of onset must then be done retrospectively, based on informant reports. However, even if the onset of certain changes was apparent to an informant at the time, recall of the timing of these changes may not be reliable. Another limitation of studies which retrospectively date onset is that they are subject to 'survivors-only bias' (Habbema and Dippell, 1986). Because all patients diagnosed at a clinic have, *ipso facto*, survived from onset to case recognition, their survival over this period will be 100%. Those cases which died between onset and recognition are not counted. Whether survivors-only bias is a problem depends on how common such early deaths are. At present, there are no relevant data available on the subject. Some researchers get around the problem of dating onset by measuring survival from the time of diagnosis (e.g. Barclay *et al.*, 1985a; Martin *et al.*, 1987a). Such measures of survival are of less theoretical interest than survival from onset. Nevertheless, survival from diagnosis is of some practical relevance to clinicians who have to advise relatives and to health-service planners.

Survival in dementing diseases is usually not studied in its own right, but in comparison with some control group. Often, the interest is in knowing whether a dementing disease reduces survival compared to the unaffected population. Some studies achieve this by selecting a matched control group (e.g. Martin *et al.*, 1987), whereas others use published life tables as the basis for comparison (e.g. Diesfeldt *et al.*, 1986). Survival studies may also compare different dementing diseases to see, for example, if survival differs between Alzheimer's disease and vascular dementia (Barclay *et al.*, 1985b; Martin *et al.*, 1987a). Another focus of interest has been in historical changes in survival. It has been claimed that dementia sufferers may now be living longer than previously and researchers have compared survival in different periods using cases from both hospital-based (Blessed and Wilson, 1982) and field studies (Rorsman *et al.*, 1985a).

3.4 COHORT STUDIES

As discussed above, an incidence study involves following a population over time and assessing the number of individuals who develop the disease under study. More generally, longitudinal studies of populations are known as cohort studies. A cohort is a group of people with a characteristic in common. Often the common characteristic is year of birth, but it could, for example, be type of occupation or place of residence. Cohort studies can be used to discover risk factors for a disease by comparing the incidence in two populations which differ in the presence or absence of the factor. For example, incidence could be calculated for the males and females in a population and compared. The ratio of the two incidence rates, I_1/I_2, is known as the **relative risk** and tells how many times higher the incidence is in one population (e.g. males) compared to the other (e.g. females). Another measure is the **attributable risk**, $I_1 - I_2$, which is simply the difference in incidence rates between the two populations. These two measures are different ways of describing the same information and either can be used, depending on what is felt to be most useful. However, the relative risk has become the more usual index, for reasons which will be discussed when dealing with case-control studies.

   To estimate the relative risk, it is not necessary that the risk factor under study be sampled as it occurs in the total population. Take, for example, a study of the effects of having a first-degree relative with Down's syndrome on the incidence of Alzheimer's disease. It would be very inefficient to do such a study using a representative sample of the general population because the number of individuals with a first-degree Down's relative would be very small. The sample size required to get enough at-risk individuals would be prohibitively large. Instead, it is possible to specifically select equal numbers of individuals with and without Down's relatives. This procedure involves considerably over-sampling the at-risk population compared to the control population.

Cohort studies of dementing diseases are fairly rare, but an example is the study by Gurland *et al.* (1983) comparing dementia in New York and London. This study found that the prevalence of dementia was higher in New York than London. Such a difference might reflect a higher incidence in New York or a longer duration of survival. However, a longitudinal follow-up revealed a higher annual incidence in New York (0.024) than in London (0.004). These incidence rates yield a relative risk of 6.0 and an attributable risk of 0.02.

Although cohort studies are, in principle, an excellent way of discovering risk factors, they have some severe practical disadvantages which mean they are seldom carried out. For a start, a cohort study necessarily takes many years to complete because the researcher has to wait for cases of the disease to develop. If a disease is rare, the incidence may be so small that very large sample sizes are required to investigate it reliably. This limitation would apply with the rarer dementing diseases and even with early-onset Alzheimer's disease. Because of the time and sample size requirements, cohort studies are generally too expensive to carry out for dementing diseases. An exception is the **historical cohort study** where existing records can be used to establish the potential risk factors and the disease incidence. In such studies, the events of interest have all occurred before the study begins. Although it is rare to have suitable existing records, very cost-efficient research can be carried out where they do exist. A good example is Mikkelsen's (1980) study in Denmark of pre-senile dementia in painters compared to bricklayers. The aim of the study was to assess whether workers exposed to organic solvents (i.e painters) are at increased risk. Membership of the two occupations was assessed by examining the files of relevant unions, while official registers of disability pensions were used to ascertain cases of pre-senile dementia. Using these existing records, Mikkelsen was able to carry out retrospectively a cohort study of 2601 painters and 1790 bricklayers, and found a relative risk of 2.0. Such a study would have been very expensive to carry out using a conventional cohort design. Another cost-efficient approach is to take cohorts originally studied for other reasons and convert them to a new purpose. Because dementing diseases primarily affect the elderly, cohort studies of younger populations which have aged are ideal for the purpose. An example is the famous Framingham study of heart disease which has now been used for the study of dementing diseases (Bachman *et al.*, 1986). A disadvantage is, of course, that the potential risk factors selected for studying heart disease may not be the ones of greatest interest for dementing diseases. Furthermore, records for assessing incidence of these diseases may be less adequate than for the diseases which were the original focus of interest. Nevertheless, the cost-efficiency of this research strategy is so great as to negate the disadvantages.

3.5 CASE-CONTROL STUDIES

Cohort studies start with groups of people differing in exposure to some potential risk factor and then follow them to assess the incidence of cases. An alternative strategy is to work backwards: identify new cases of the dementing disease and compare them with controls in terms of exposure to potential risk factors. Such studies are known as case-control studies, and are a far more economical way of establishing risk factors. Unlike cohort studies, case-control studies do not require longitudinal follow-up and are feasible with diseases which have a very low incidence.

3.5.1 Measuring risk

Although they have advantages of economy, case-control studies do not yield the range of information provided by cohort studies. They cannot be used to estimate incidence rates or measures derived from incidence such as the attributable risk and relative risk. What they do yield is an **odds ratio**. If a population contains d cases of a disease and n non-cases, then the odds of disease are d/n. If two groups are compared (e.g. cases and controls), an odds ratio (OR) can be calculated.

$$OR = \frac{d_1/n_1}{d_2/n_2}$$

With rare diseases, this measure is an approximation to the relative risk. In practice, the incidence of a disease has to be quite high (e.g. greater than 0.1 per year) for the odds ratio to be a poor approximation to the relative risk. Alzheimer's disease, which is the most common of the dementing diseases, would satisfy the rare disease assumption, even amongst the very elderly. It is perhaps because case-control studies can yield an approximation to the relative risk that this index of risk has proved more popular than the attributable risk.

   Table 3.2 illustrates the calculation of an odds ratio using data taken from a case-control study by Axelson *et al.* (1976). This study took cases of neuropsychiatric disorders from a Swedish pension fund register and compared them to controls from the same register. The cases and controls were compared on occupational exposure to solvents. The table shows the data on pre-senile and senile dementia only. Amongst exposed individuals the odds of disease was 7/35, compared to 17/213 for non-exposed individuals. This gives an odds ratio of (7/35)/(17/213) =

Table 3.2 Example of calculation of an odds ratio using data from Axelson *et al.* (1976)

	No. exposed to solvents	No. not exposed	Odds of exposure
Dementia cases	7	17	7/17
Controls	35	213	35/213
Odds of disease	7/35	17/213	

$$\text{Odds ratio (OR)} = \frac{7/35}{17/213} = \frac{0.20}{0.08} = 2.5$$

2.5. It is interesting that the same answer could have been derived by comparing the odds of exposure rather than odds of disease: (7/17)/(35/213) = 2.5. In other words, the odds ratio gives both the increase in odds of exposure amongst diseased individuals as well as the increase in odds of disease amongst exposed individuals.

3.5.2 Selecting cases and controls

The basic strategy behind a case-control study is to collect a representative sample of incident cases from a population and compare them to a representative sample of non-cases from the same population. The cases must be incident (i.e. new), rather than prevalent, or else there will be an over-representation of cases who survive longer. Some of the risk factors revealed by a study of prevalent cases might relate to risk for survival after developing the disease, rather than risk of developing the disease *per se*.

As discussed before, the point at which a case becomes incident is difficult to define with dementing diseases. In case-control studies, cases are usually incident as far as formal medical recognition is concerned, but cognitive deterioration may have been present for quite some time before that. Cases which do not survive to formal recognition will be excluded and, to this extent, some survivors-only bias will be present. However, the more important source of bias in case-control studies is case-ascertainment bias. Those cases not recognized by treating physicians will be excluded. With pre-senile dementias, it is likely that most cases will be recognized, but senile dementia cases may go unrecognized by treating physicians. Community surveys of dementia in Britain and West Germany have shown that primary-care physicians miss a large percentage of cases (Williamson *et al.*, 1964; Parsons, 1965; Weyerer, 1983; O'Connor *et al.*, 1988). If detected and non-detected cases differ in the potential risk factors under investigation, then

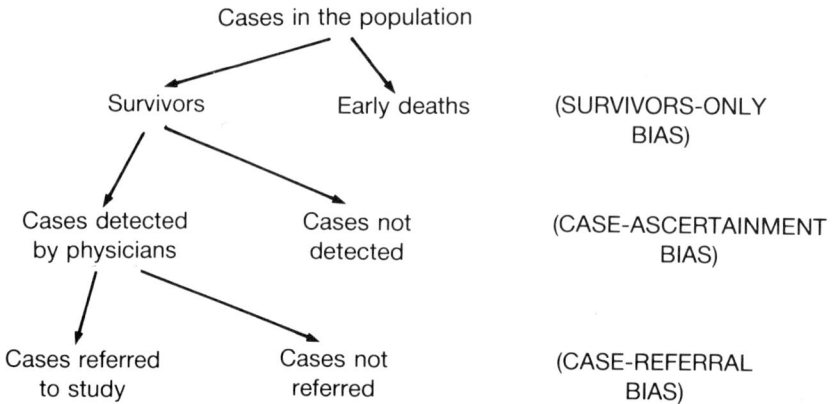

Figure 3.1   Biases that can arise in case selection in a case-control study.

spurious effects may arise. Once cases in a population are detected, they must all be referred to the study. If treating physicians fail to refer some cases because, for example, they are too frail or their family show a lack of interest in the study, further bias could be introduced. Figure 3.1 shows the process that cases in the population have to go through before being recruited to a case-control study, and the biases that can arise along the way.

Control selection is, in many ways, more difficult than case selection. Controls should come from the same defined population as cases. In practice, the population under study is often not clearly specified by researchers, but can be defined by tracing back the process by which cases come to be included in the study. For example, if cases come from the population of potential attenders at certain neurological clinics, then controls should come from the same population. If exclusion criteria are not applied equally to cases and controls, spurious associations may result, as in the case-control study of Alzheimer's disease by Heyman *et al.* (1984) in which a higher frequency of hypertension was found in controls than cases. On the surface, this would indicate that hypertension is a protection factor for Alzheimer's disease, but the association was an artefact due to exclusion of cases with hypertension, but not controls with hypertension.

In an attempt to make controls as comparable as possible to cases, case-control studies of dementing diseases generally match cases and controls in pairs on variables like age, sex or area of residence. Without matching, cases may be very different on some variables which are of little interest. For example, with dementing diseases, a strictly random selection strategy would lead to cases being mainly elderly and controls much younger. This difference would reflect the fact that age is a genuine risk factor, but researchers are generally not interested in knowing this. While the effects of variables like age can be removed during the statistical analysis, matching is probably a simpler strategy. While matching is often useful, it can be carried too far if cases and controls are either directly or indirectly matched on potential risk factors. This sort of problem is referred to as 'over-matching'. As an example, imagine that exposure to some industrial chemical is a risk factor for Alzheimer's disease, but occurs much more commonly in lower socio-economic groups. If cases and controls were matched for socio-economic status, the strength of the relationship between the exposure and Alzheimer's disease would be artifically reduced.

Matching of cases and controls in pairs also effects the calculation of the odds ratio. It is simply calculated from the numbers of pairs discordant on the risk factor. For example, in Chandra *et al.*'s (1987a) case-control study of Alzheimer's disease, there were 64 matched pairs of subjects. When head trauma was examined as a potential risk factor, there were six pairs where the case had head trauma and the control did not, but only one pair where the control had head trauma and the

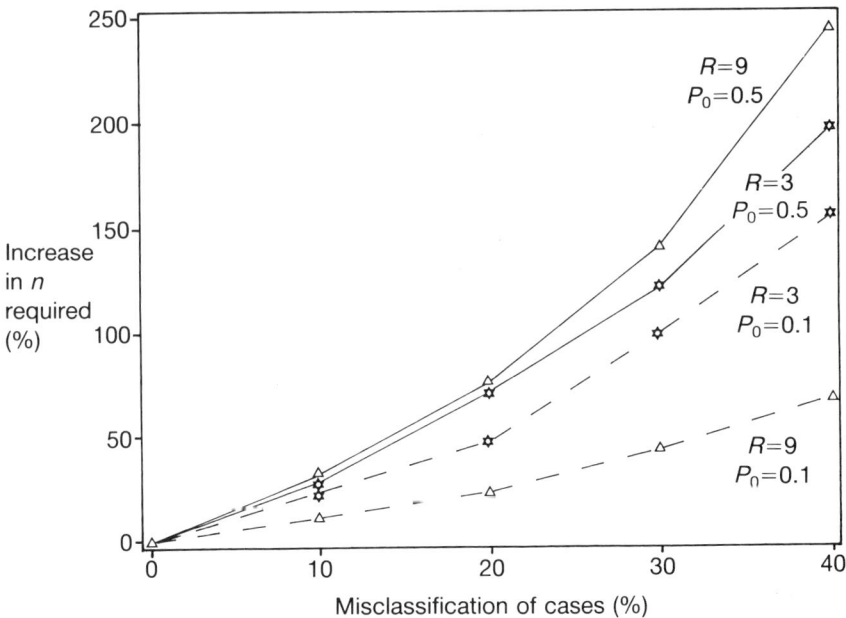

Figure 3.2 Percentage increase in number of subjects required for case-control studies as a function of misclassification of cases ($\alpha = 0.05$, $\beta = 0.10$, 2-tailed). Adapted from Henderson and Jorm (1987).

case did not. The odds ratio is calculated by dividing the two counts of discordant pairs: $6/1 = 6.0$.

As far as case diagnosis is concerned, case-control studies have considerable advantages over community surveys because they are generally based around clinics and extensive assessment is possible. Nevertheless, case-control studies of dementing disorders are usually carried out on clinically diagnosed cases without neuropathological confirmation. With clinical diagnosis, there will inevitably be some error, so that some cases will be false positives. With clinically diagnosed Alzheimer's disease, diagnostic error of up to 20% is possible, even with thorough assessment (Sulkava *et al.*, 1983; Mölsa *et al.*, 1985). A similar level of inaccuracy applies to the clinical diagnosis of vascular dementia (Mölsa *et al.*, 1985; Erkinjuntti *et al.*, 1988). The effect of including misclassifications in the case group is to weaken the strength of any associations found. In planning a case-control study, the researcher must choose a sample size which is sufficiently large to detect any effects likely to be present. Schlesselman (1982) has given statistical power tables which show the sample size required to detect a particular level of relative risk where one has an estimate of the frequency of exposure to a risk factor in the control group. The effect of contaminating the case group with a proportion of controls is to increase the number of subjects required to detect a particular relative risk. Figure 3.2 shows the percentage increase required in sample size at different misclassification rates. The increase required is influenced by the exposure rate (P_0) and relative risk (R) associated with the risk factor under study. It can be seen that the increase in required sample size may be considerable, even for misclassification rates as low as 20%. Consequently, case-control studies of clincially diagnosed dementing disorders must use larger sample sizes than would be required if perfect diagnostic accuracy were assumed.

There are two types of control groups which have proved popular in studies of dementing diseases: hospital controls and community controls. Hospital controls are selected from non-demented patients attending the same hospital as the cases. This type of control group is used on the rationale that cases are selected from the population of hospital attenders, so controls should be as well. Although in principle straightforward, there can be practical difficulties with hospital controls. Such controls are attending the hospital for other diseases which have their own risk factors. It is important to ensure that any risk factors found to differentiate cases and controls are not, in fact, protection factors for the controls' disease. Conversely, if both cases and controls have diseases with common risk factors, the effect would be masked by the higher exposure rates in controls as well as cases. For such reasons, it would be unwise to take controls who all have one type of non-dementing disease. The usual strategy is to take controls with a variety of diseases, hoping that any potentially artifactual effects will cancel out. Also, any diseases with known risk factors or protection factors in common with the dementing disease can be avoided.

Community controls would seem to obviate these problems, but have others of their own. Such controls are used on the assumption that they are drawn from the same community population as the cases. However, cases enrolled in a case-control study are likely to be only a subset of all incident cases in the community. For example, Heyman *et al.* (1984) found that their cases were significantly better educated than their community controls, which they attributed to a selection bias for cases enrolling in the study. In other words, less-educated cases tended not to enrol in the study. There may also be considerable problems in recruiting community controls because they are less likely to be co-operative with a research study than hospital controls. Those who co-operate with the study may be different from the refusers, leading to spurious differences between cases and controls. If matching is attempted on variables like age, sex and area of residence, the problem of finding suitable community controls is even greater because of the more limited range of possible subjects. Because of the problems inherent with both hospital and community controls, some researchers have used both in the same study (e.g. French *et al.*, 1985; Amaducci *et al.*, 1986). If contradictory results arise with the two control groups, the researcher must consider possible sources of bias in each group which could have produced the discrepancy.

3.5.3 Assessment of risk factors

Case-control studies proceed from disease to risk factors, rather than the other way round, so assessment of exposures is necessarily retrospective. The usual method of assessing potential risk factors in a case-control study is to interview cases and controls. Usually, risk factor interviews involve asking subjects about the frequency or date of certain events in the past. It is assumed that this information is accurately stored in the subject's memory and can be retrieved. However, research into autobio-graphical questions of the sort used in surveys shows that quite complex cognitive processes are involved in answering such questions and the answers can often be inaccurate (Bradburn *et al.*, 1987). For example, when subjects are asked how often they have visited the doctor in the past five years, they do not simply retrieve all the visits from memory and add them up. Rather, they base their answer on inferences. For example, they may recall the number of visits in the past half year and multiply by 10, on the assumption that the rate of visits is stable over time. There are also problems in dating past events. If, for example, a subject is asked for the date of an operation, the exact year may not be stored in memory, but may be reconstructed by reference to landmark autobiographical events e.g. 'It was after my first grandchild was born, so it must have been around 1970'. Inferences of this type can lead to considerable inaccuracies, but these can be minimized by framing questions in the light of an understanding of human memory limitations.

With dementing diseases, the problem of accurate memory retrieval is even greater because the disorders under investigation involve memory impairment. In order to circumvent the poor memories of cases, informants are used. Although controls may provide more valid information, they must be treated the same way as cases, so informants are used for them as well. Although it is generally impossible to check the reliability of recall for the informants of cases, this can be done for the informants of controls by comparing their reports to those of the controls themselves. Heyman *et al.* (1984) have reported control/informant agreement for a number of illnesses, accidents, medical treatments and family characteristics. The degree of agreement varied considerably, being very low for influenza during World War I, lung disease, liver disease, contact with wildlife and family history of dementing illness, but very high for myocardial infarction, diabetes, use of analgesics, diabetic medications and hypertensive/cardiac medications. Although the poor agreement on events of long ago (e.g. influenza during World War I) is not surprising, the results for many of the other potential risk factors are not easily explained. Rocca *et al.* (1986) have similarly reported on agreement between informants and controls, but found that it was fairly good, there being over 80% agreement for 45 of the 57 tested items. Agreement was poorest for questions dealing with antacid drug use, number of cigarettes smoked per day, and number of jobs held. The effect of unreliability in informant reports is to make any true risk factors harder to detect and constitutes an important problem for case-control studies of dementing diseases.

To help overcome limitations of recall, some researchers have advocated the use of multiple informants with expertise on different parts of the subject's lifespan (Anthony, 1988). For example, Pickle *et al.* (1983) found that spouses and children were more able to give responses about the subject's adult life, while siblings could more often answer questions about family characteristics and early life. Another commonly-used method of increasing the validity of informant reports is to ask them to gather relevant records before the interview takes place. However, this does not necessarily guarantee accuracy. Bradburn *et al.* (1987) cite Dutch research showing that only 47% of respondents who consulted records gave the correct balance in their bank account – an unimpressive rise over the 31% who were correct without records.

Because recall of past events frequently involves inferences, rather than direct retrieval of those events from memory, informants may be influenced by knowledge of the purpose of the case-control study. Thus, if informants know a study is about dementia, they may be more liable to report information which seems plausible in light of the diagnosis. For example, previous diseases and injuries involving the brain and family history of dementing diseases might seem to make sense in light of the patient's present condition. Unfortunately, there is no information available on what the general public regard as plausible risk factors for dementing disorders or whether such expectations influence recall. Nevertheless, some case-control studies have taken the precaution of keeping informants blind as to the purpose of the study (French *et al.*, 1985; Chandra *et al.*, 1987a). It is also possible that interviewers could probe more deeply on certain factors if they know the purpose of the study, so they have also been kept blind in these studies.

One method of assessing whether recall bias is operating is to include people with another type of dementing disease as an additional control group. Thus, in a case-control study of Alzheimer's disease, a control group of vascular dementia cases could be used as well as the normal control group. If informants are biased towards recalling events which could be plausible causes of the dementia, they will show this for both dementing diseases. It could of course be possible that both types of dementing disease share a common risk factor, but if an association emerges for one disease but not the other, recall bias becomes a less plausible explanation.

3.5.4 Drawing causal inferences

Case-control studies are capable of assessing associations between risk factors and diseases. Usually, however, researchers wish to know whether the observed associations are of aetiological significance. Associations can arise in several ways other than through a direct causal link. One possibility is that the factor associated with the disease is an effect rather than a cause. Although case-control studies deal with incident cases, these are only incident to a particular degree of severity, or to a particular stage of case recognition. Cases may have undergone years of cognitive decline before being enrolled in a study. Thus, any associations between the disease and factors in the recent past may reflect early effects of the disease. An example of this ambiguity is Erkinjuntti *et al.*'s (1987a) study showing that a history of snoring is more common in cases of both Alzheimer's disease and vascular dementia than in controls. This association may have arisen as an effect of the dementing diseases or it may have been an antecedent. Unless a risk factor can be shown to be present many years before case ascertainment, the possibility of it being a disease effect must be considered.

Another way a non-causal association can arise is for a risk factor to be correlated with another factor which is responsible for the disease association. An association between socio-economic status and a dementing disease might be of this sort. Socio-economic status could not directly cause a disease in itself, but might be correlated with lifestyle factors and occupational exposures which are causally related. If an association is only a proxy for a causal relationship with some other variable, then the real association is likely to be even larger than the proxy one. Accordingly, some authorities argue that a large relative risk is less likely to be due to some other variable than is a small relative risk (Schlesselman, 1982).

Where there are two inter-related risk factors for a disease, it is possible to test theories of causal priority by holding one variable constant and seeing whether the other is still associated with the disease. An example of this strategy occurred in the case-control study of Alzheimer's disease by French *et al.* (1985) which found that head trauma was a risk factor. Subsequently, Rimm (1986) pointed out that the controls included more widows than the cases. If spouse informants were more likely to recall accurately an incident of head trauma than other relatives, the difference between cases and controls may have emerged for this reason. French *et al.* (1986) tested this possibility by re-analysing the data for cases and controls who had a spouse informant. When type of informant was not controlled, the odds ratios were 4.5 using hospital controls and 2.8 using neighbourhood controls. With spouse informants only, the odds ratios actually increased to 9.0 and 12.0 respectively. The data thus supported the theory that head trauma is a cause of Alzheimer's disease better than the alternative that cases tend to have different types of informants who better recalled incidents of head trauma. Reasoning of this sort can never establish causality, but can help bolster the case by ruling out competing accounts of the association.

The aetiology of most dementing diseases is unlikely to be simple. Rather than there being a single causal factor, such as a gene or an environmental toxin, there is likely to be an interplay of factors. Sometimes these factors may have independent additive effects, as when both a gene and an environmental toxin increase risk for the disease. However, in some cases there may be interaction effects, so that one factor magnifies another. Thus, an environmental toxin might only have an effect where there is host susceptibility, such as the presence of a predisposing gene. Neither the toxin nor the gene are sufficient in themselves to produce the disease, but do so in combination. Less extreme interaction effects are possible. For example, the toxin might increase the risk for the disease whether or not the gene is present, but its effects are greater with the gene. Case-control studies can be used to assess interaction effects between risk factors of this sort, but require much greater sample sizes than for assessing independent effects.

Although case-control and cohort studies can give useful clues to causal relationships, they are incapable of firmly establishing causality. This can only be clearly established through experimental studies in which the hypothesized aetiological factor is systematically varied and all other factors are held constant. If varying this factor increases or decreases incidence of the disease, then its causal status is clear. In practice, experimental studies of this type are rarely possible except on animals. An exception is the experimental evaluation of preventive programmes in which risk factors are reduced in an effort to prevent a disease. Knowledge of dementing diseases is presently too rudimentary for such preventive trials to be attempted. However, if the epidemiological study of dementing diseases is to be of practical value, successful prevention will one day be demonstrated.

3.6 RESEARCH INTEGRATION

Epidemiological research on dementing disorders is growing at a rapid rate. Already there are specific topics on which more than 60 studies have been published (e.g. the prevalence of dementia) and a similar situation will soon prevail with other topics. When the literature on an issue becomes large, it can become quite difficult to draw any clear conclusions, particularly if the studies involve diverse methods and have apparently conflicting conclusions. The traditional method of integrating information from a large number of studies is the **narrative literature review**. This involves the reviewer describing all the studies and attempting to come up with some sort of interpretive synthesis. The cognitive processes by which reviewers achieve this integration are poorly understood, but probably have much in common with the descriptive–interpretive approaches to primary research used in disciplines like history, literary criticism and social anthropology. It is ironic that epidemiological researchers who use quantitative techniques to analyse their primary data typically turn to quite a different methodology when attempting secondary synthesis of studies.

A limitation of many narrative literature reviews is that they over-emphasize the statistical significance or non-significance of individual studies. Thus, if 20 studies have been carried out on the same issue, and four of these produced statistically significant results, many reviewers would conclude that there is no association because the other 16 studies produced negative results. However, only one significant result would be expected by chance out of 20 studies. A real effect may well exist even if most of the studies are non-significant. The size of the effect may be too small to produce consistently significant results unless very large sample sizes are used.

The alternative to the narrative literature review is **meta-analysis**. This approach involves the application of quantitative scoring and statistical analysis to research integration. In a meta-analysis, the reviewer reads each study and codes its attributes in a quantitative manner. The coded characteristics might include: sample size, sampling procedure, country where the research was carried out, method of diagnosis, age and sex composition of the sample, and effect size (incidence rate, prevalence rate, relative risk). These coded characteristics are then analysed using conventional statistical procedures, with the individual study being the unit of analysis. Data from sets of homogeneous studies can be pooled to arrive at summary statistics for the size of various effects. Meta-analysis has become increasingly popular as a method of research integration in the social and behavioural sciences and its use is now spreading to epidemiology and public health (Louis *et al.*, 1985; Greenland, 1987).

Meta-analytic techniques can potentially be applied to the integration of epidemiological research of almost any type: prevalence, incidence, mortality or risk factor studies. However, as yet these techniques have been little used to integrate research on dementing diseases. An exception is Jorm *et al.*'s (1987) meta-analysis of dementia prevalence studies which showed that prevalence rises exponentially with age. Similar analysis techniques to the ones they used could potentially be applied to incidence or mortality. The integration of risk factor research is another area where meta-analytic techniques could be used. Greenland (1987) and Walker *et al.* (1988) have proposed methods for this purpose. With Greenland's method, studies are coded in terms of type of design (e.g. case-control vs. cohort), exposures examined, possible confounders and moderating variables, and effect sizes found. Effect size is quantified in terms of relative risk. The aim of the meta-analysis is to discover whether there is heterogeneity in effects across studies and, if so, what variables could account for this (e.g. differences in design). If results of studies are fairly homogeneous in effect size, they can be weighted according to standard error of measurement and pooled to arrive at a summary estimate of relative risk. In Walker *et al.*'s (1988) approach to meta-analysis, relative risks and their associated confidence intervals are graphed for each study of a particular risk factor. Areas of overlap among confidence intervals from this set of studies can be used to derive a summary confidence interval for the risk factor. In an application of meta-analysis to risk factors for Alzheimer's disease, Mortimer (1989) has used data from a number of case-control studies. He produced summary odds ratios for various exposures by pooling data across the studies.

Comparison of relative risks or odds ratios across different studies may present problems, however, for a disorder like Alzheimer's disease where different cut-offs may be used to separate diseased from non-diseased individuals (Jorm, 1989). Imagine, for example, that the cut-off for defining a case of Alzheimer's disease was varied so as to produce two different definitions of a case. The effect would be to make incidence rates higher under one definition than the other. If the more liberal cut-off made incidence k times higher in both exposed and non-exposed individuals, then estimates of relative risk would be unaffected because the multiplicative factor (k) would occur on both the numerator and denominator of the relative risk and cancel out, i.e. $I_1/I_2 = kI_1/kI_2$. If, however, varying cut-offs had an additive (or any but multiplicative) effect on incidence rates, then relative risks derived using different cut-offs would not be comparable, i.e. $I_1/I_2 \neq (I_1 + k)/(I_2 + k)$. Whether varying the cut-off to define a case has a consistently multiplicative effect on incidence rates is unknown, but has important implications for any attempt to integrate data across studies. Such a problem would not arise with a disease for which cases and non-cases could be consistently defined across studies.

3.7 CONCLUSION

Epidemiological research methods were originally developed for infectious diseases and only later extended to chronic diseases of ageing. The major dementing diseases are in many ways different from infectious diseases, giving rise to problems in the direct application of these research methods. These problems spring chiefly from the difficulty in dividing the population into categorically distinct groups of cases and non-cases.

4 Prevalence

Prevalence has arguably been the most researched topic in the epidemiology of dementing diseases. There are currently over 60 studies of prevalence in general population samples. These studies vary in the degree of their diagnostic specificity. One type of study looks at the prevalence of cognitive impairment, with a high score on a cognitive screening test being used to define a case. Although most cases of cognitive impairment will be due to dementia, there will be poorly educated, mentally retarded and learning disabled individuals as well. Such studies are, however, a minority. The majority of prevalence studies ascertain cases of the dementia syndrome, without attempting diagnosis of specific dementing diseases. In the older studies, rigorous diagnostic criteria for dementia were not available and assessment was often rudimentary, so that in practice these sometimes dealt with cognitive impairment rather than dementia. It is often difficult in retrospect to determine whether a study is best regarded as having ascertained cognitive impairment or dementia. Finally, there are the studies which attempted clinical diagnoses of specific dementing diseases, usually Alzheimer's disease and vascular dementia, these being the most prevalent dementias. Table 4.1 lists the studies since 1945 estimating the prevalence of either the dementia syndrome or cognitive impairment, while Table 4.2 gives the prevalence studies attempting clinical diagnosis of specific dementing diseases.

4.1 PROBLEMS WITH THE INTEGRATION OF PREVALENCE STUDIES

With such a lot of data available, it might be expected that some quite definite conclusions could be drawn about the prevalence of dementing diseases. However, integration of these data has proven difficult because of the great diversity of methods used in these studies.

Some reviewers of the dementia prevalence literature have concluded that the research is too diverse to permit meaningful integration. For example, Gunner-Svensson and Jensen (1976) did a thorough review of nine prevalence studies from Scandinavia and Britain. They concluded that 'comparison of the various results is difficult as most of the authors have not intended their investigations for mutual comparison. It is clear that there are many dissimilarities in the milieus involved, in the methods used, in the prerequisites of the interviewers and assessors, and in the classification of the results' (p. 283). Gunner-Svensson and Jensen saw integration of results as being possible in the future if different investigators were to use standardized methods. Some progress towards standardization has occurred in the decade after their review, e.g. the US/UK study (Gurland *et al.*, 1983), and the Epidemiologic Catchment Area studies in the US (Myers *et al.*, 1984). However, studies using a standard replicable methodology are still far from the norm.

A more recent review by Henderson and Kay (1984) reached similar conclusions about the lack of comparability of prevalence studies. They reviewed the results from twelve studies which, they concluded, could only be looked upon 'as an assembly of rather disparate measures' (p. 59) because of the great variation in methodological characteristics. Henderson and Kay listed a number of variations in method which could influence the prevalence rates found.

1. *The size of the sample.* Large samples will permit more accurate estimates of prevalence than smaller ones. However, as the sample size becomes larger, the resources available for case ascertainment may be spread thinner and some cases consequently missed.
2. *The sample composition.* Some studies include only individuals living in the community, while others involve institutional residents as well. Although the proportion of the population in institutional care is small, the prevalence of dementia is invariably high in this group.
3. *The age ranges covered.* Most studies estimate prevalence for the elderly as a group. While in many studies the elderly are defined as aged 65+, in other studies they are defined as 60+ or 70+.
4. *The proportion of very old in the denominator.* Even prevalence rates for those aged 65+ cannot easily be compared across studies because the age structure within the elderly group may differ across populations. Some elderly populations will have a greater proportion who are very elderly (e.g. aged 80+). Because dementia prevalence increases with age, the proportion who are very elderly will affect the crude prevalence rate for the elderly as an overall group. To overcome this problem, it is necessary to report age-specific prevalence rates, but this requires large sample sizes.
5. *The method for identifying cases.* Some studies use personal interviews of all subjects, while others use a case register or key informants to detect cases.
6. *The content of the interview.* Interviews may be by clinicians using their own unstructured examinations (particularly in the older studies) or may involve standardized clinical interviews. While standardized interviews are clearly preferable, there are considerable differences in their content and in the qualifications of the people who may use them.

Table 4.1 Prevalence studies of (non-specific) dementia or cognitive impairment

Author(s) and year	Country	Age range of elderly	Age-specific rates available	Terminology
Ben-Arie et al. (1983)	South Africa	65+	No	Dementia
Bentsen (1970)	Norway	60+	No	Vascular and senile psychosis
Bland et al. (1988)	Canada	65+	Yes	Cognitive impairment
Bond (1987)	Britain	65+	Yes	Organic disorder
Bremer (1951)	Norway	60+	Yes	Senile psychosis
Campbell et al. (1983)	New Zealand	65+	Yes	Dementia
Clarke et al. (1986)	Britain	75+	Yes	Cognitive impairment
Cooper (1984)	West Germany	65+	No	Senile and arteriosclerotic dementia
Engedal et al. (1988)	Norway	75+	Yes	Dementia
Essen-Möller et al. (1956)	Sweden	60+	Yes	Senile and arteriosclotic deterioration
Gilmore (1974)	Britain	65+	No	Dementia
Griffiths et al. (1987)	Britain	60+	Yes	Dementia
Gruenberg (1961)	USA	65+	Yes	Certifiable
Gruer et al. (1975)	Britain	65+	Yes	Chronic brain syndrome
Hagnell et al (1981)	Sweden	60+	Yes	Age psychosis
Ichinowatari et al. (1987)	Japan	65+	Yes	Dementia
Jensen (1963)	Denmark	65+	No	Senile dementia
Jensen and Polloi (1988)	Palau	90+	No	Dementia

Study	Country	Age		Diagnosis
Kato (1969)	Japan	60+	No	Organic psychosis
Kay et al. (1985)	Australia	70+	Yes	Dementia
Kidson (1967)	Australia	60+	No	Dementia
Leighton et al. (1963)	Canada	60+	Yes	Senility
Lin (1953)	Taiwan	60+	Yes	Senile psychosis
Lin et al. (1969)	Taiwan	61+	Yes	Senile psychosis
Magnusson and Helgason (1981)	Iceland	74–76, 80–82	Yes	Senile, vascular and mixed dementias
Maule et al. (1984)	Britain	62+	Yes	Chronic brain syndrome
Morgan et al. (1987)	Britain	65+	Yes	Cognitive impairment
Mowry and Burvill (1988)	Australia	70+	Yes	Dementia
Myers et al. (1984)	Britain	65+	No	Cognitive impairment
Nielsen (1962)	Denmark	65+	Yes	Senile dementia
Nielsen et al. (1982)	Denmark	70+	Yes	Senile dementia
Nilsson and Persson (1984)	Sweden	70, 75, 79	Yes	Dementia
Park and Ha (1988)	South Korea	65+	Yes	Cognitive impairment
Parsons (1965)	Britain	65+	No	Serious dementia
Pasamanick et al. (1957)	USA	65+	No	Unspecified psychosis
Primrose (1962)	Britain	65+	No	Senile, arteriosclerotic and mixed dementias
Robertson et al. (1984)	Canada	65+	No	Dementia
Sheldon (1948)	Britain	65+	Yes	Definite mental failure, demented
Weissman et al. (1985)	USA	65+	Yes	Cognitive impairment
Weyerer (1983)	West Germany	65+	No	Senile dementia
Yu et al. (1989)	China	55+	Yes	Cognitive impairment

Table 4.2 Prevalence studies of specific dementing diseases (Alzheimer and vascular dementias)

Author(s) and year	Country	Age range rates available	Age-specific	Terminology
Åkesson (1969)	Sweden	65+	Yes	Senile and arteriosclerotic psychoses
Bollerup (1975)	Denmark	70	Only one age	Senile and arteriosclerotic dementias
Brayne and Calloway (1989)	Britain	70–79	Yes	Senile dementia of Alzheimer type and multi-infarct dementia
Broe et al. (1976)	Britain	65+	Yes	Vascular and senile dementias
Chen (1987)	China	60+	No	Senile and vascular dementias
D'Alessandro et al. (1988)	San Marino	66+	Yes	Primary degenerative, chronic progressive and secondary (incl. multi-infarct) dementias
Evans et al. (1989)	USA	65+	Yes	Alzheimer's disease and multi-infarct dementia
Folstein et al. (1985)	USA	65+	No	Alzheimer's disease and multi-infarct dementia
Gavrilova (1984)	USSR	60+	No	Senile and vascular dementias
Gavrilova et al. (1987)	USSR	60+	Yes	Senile and vascular dementias
Gurland et al. (1983)	Britain	65+	No	Alzheimer and arteriosclerotic dementias
Gurland et al. (1983)	USA	65+	No	Alzheimer and arteriosclerotic dementias
Hasegawa et al. (1983)	Japan	65+	Yes	Senile and multi-infarct dementias
Hasegawa et al. (1986)	Japan	65+	Yes	Senile and vascular dementias
Kaneko (1975)	Japan	65+	Yes	Senile and vascular dementias

Study	Country	Age		Type of dementia
Kaneko (1975)	Japan	60+	Yes	Senile and vascular dementias
Karasawa et al. (1982)	Japan	65+	Yes	Senile and vascular dementias
Kay et al. (1964a)	Britain	65+	Yes	Senile and arteriosclerotic organic brain syndromes
Kokmen et al. (1989)	USA	65+	Yes	Alzheimer's disease and all dementias
Kuang and Zhao (1984)	China	60+	No	Vascular dementia and senility from age
Li et al. (1989)	China	60+	Yes	Multi-infarct and primary degenerative dementias
Lippi et al. (1989)	Italy	60+	Yes	Alzheimer's disease and multi-infarct dementia
Makiya (1978)	Japan	60+	No	Senile and multi-infarct dementias
Mölsa et al. (1982)	Finland	65+	Yes	Senile dementia and dementia with associated arteriosclerosis
Motohiro et al. (1985)	Japan	65+	Yes	Senile and multi-infarct dementias
O'Connor et al. (1989c)	Britain	75+	Yes	Senile dementia of Alzheimer's type and vascular dementia
Pinessi et al. (1984)	Italy	65+	Yes	Dementias of Alzheimer and vascular types
Rorsman et al. (1986)	Sweden	60+	Yes	Senile and multi-infarct dementias
Schoenberg et al. (1985)	USA	60+	Yes	Primary chronic progressive dementia
Shibayama et al. (1986)	Japan	65+	No	Multi-infarct dementia and senile dementia of Alzheimer type
Sternberg and Gawrilowa (1978)	USSR	60+	Yes	Vascular and senile psychoses
Sulkava et al. (1985a)	Finland	65+	Yes	Primary degenerative and vascular dementias
Zhao (1986)	China	60+	No	Senile and multi-infarct dementias

7. *The use of supplementary diagnostic information.* Some studies involve only interviews with subjects, while others supplement this with informant data. There is also variable use of laboratory tests and brain scans to aid diagnosis.

8. *The diagnostic criteria used.* Many of the early studies used idiosyncratic diagnostic criteria. The advent of standardized diagnostic criteria has helped considerably, but even these may be interpreted differently by different researchers. Computerized diagnostic algorithms used in harness with standardized interviews are the ideal solution, but are used in few studies. A particular source of variation in diagnostic practice is the grading of dementia severity. Although descriptions like mild, moderate and severe are commonly used, there may be little consistency across investigators in the degree of impairment these descriptors are used to refer to.

9. *The type of prevalence estimate.* Most studies estimate point prevalence, but studies estimating period prevalence are not unknown. However, with a low-incidence chronic disease, the difference between point prevalence and, say, one-year period prevalence may not be too great.

Like Gunner-Svensson and Jensen (1976), Henderson and Kay argued that it may be possible in the future to look for real differences in prevalence between populations, but this will only become possible if prevalence estimates are not biased by substantial differences in methods.

4.2 INTEGRATIVE CONCLUSIONS ABOUT PREVALENCE

Other reviewers of the dementia prevalence literature have been less pessimistic about the possibility of drawing generalizable conclusions. For example, Kay and Bergmann (1980) regarded the results of studies by Nielsen (1962), Kay *et al.* (1970) and Kaneko (1975) as being sufficiently similar to be pooled together to arrive at more stable age-specific prevalence rates for moderate-to-severe dementia. Their summary rates are shown in Table 4.3. However, Kay and Bergmann felt that the prevalence rates for mild dementia were quite variable, suggesting that there were different concepts of mild dementia across investigators. More recently, Ineichen (1987) has concluded that Kay and Bergmann's (1980) figures were too high, because research since their review has reported lower rates. Accordingly, he has adjusted these downwards to arrive at 'rule-of-thumb' prevalence estimates of 1% for 65–74-year-olds and 10% for those aged 75+.

Other attempts to summarize the prevalence literature have used more sophisticated statistical approaches. Preston (1986) derived a formula for age-specific prevalence rates using data from a study by Campbell *et al.* (1983) in New Zealand. The Campbell *et al.* data were

Table 4.3 Prevalence rates (%) of dementia derived by Kay and Bergman (1980) from three studies

Age group	Male prevalence (SE)	Female prevalence (SE)	Both sexes
65–69	3.9 (± 0.97)	0.5 (± 0.35)	2.1
70–74	4.1 (± 1.21)	2.7 (± 0.85)	3.3
75–79	8.0 (± 1.99)	7.9 (± 1.67)	8.0
80+	13.2 (± 2.64)	20.9 (± 2.68)	17.7

used because their sample was weighted towards the older age groups which have the highest prevalence of dementia. Furthermore, the study yielded more cases of dementia than had previous studies. It was therefore possible to arrive at more stable age-specific prevalence estimates from this study than from its predecessors. Preston (1986) used regression techniques to arrive at the formula:

$$P = \exp(-12.2041 + 0.1258X)$$

where P = probability of dementia for individuals aged between X and

$X + 5$ years; and X = age in years.

According to this formula, the prevalence rate of dementia (P) rises exponentially with age (X). Application of the formula yields the age-specific prevalence rates shown in Table 4.4. As would be expected, Preston's exponential formula gives a good fit to the data from which it is derived. However, Preston also evaluated the fit of the formula to age-specific prevalence data from studies by Essen-Möller (1956), Primrose (1962), Nielsen (1962), Kaneko (1975) and Kay *et al.* (1970). In all cases he found that the observed number of dementia cases did not depart significantly from the number expected by the formula. However, the

Table 4.4 Age-specific prevalence rates (%) derived from Preston's (1986) formula

Age group	Prevalence rate
65–69	1.8
70–74	3.3
75–79	6.3
80–84	11.7
85–89	22.0
90+	41.3

95% confidence interval for the formula is so wide that only large departures would reach statistical significance. The large confidence interval results because the formula was based on only a single study.

Jorm *et al.* (1987) later developed a statistical model of age-specific prevalence using data from all published studies, rather than just one as had Preston (1986). They located 22 studies published between 1945 and 1985 which gave usable age-specific data. Jorm *et al.* attempted to resolve empirically the issue of whether methodological differences are a source of variation in prevalence rates by a meta-analysis of published studies. It was possible to code the methodological features of each study and correlate these with reported prevalence rates. If method-ological differences contribute to variation in prevalence rates, then some correlations would be expected. Indeed, the 22 studies were found to yield significantly different prevalence rates and virtually all the methodological variables which could be coded from the studies had a significant effect on the reported rates. For example, studies using a broad definition of dementia (e.g. including all cognitive impairment) had rates 64% higher than those using a more narrow definition. In view of the significant differences between studies, it was not possible to derive a simple formula for age-specific prevalence as Preston (1986) had attempted. Instead, Jorm *et al.* (1987) proposed the following exponential statistical model.

$$P_i = \exp (S_i - 13.50 + 0.137X)$$

where P_i = probability of dementia for individuals age X years from study i; S_i = variable 'study' term, specific to study i, but independent of age; and X = age in years.

It is instructive to compare this statistical model with Preston's formula. They both describe an exponential rise in prevalence with age, but Jorm *et al.*'s (1987) model says that the actual rates differ from study to study by a multiplicative factor, $\exp (S_i)$. According to the model, prevalence doubles with every 5.1 years of age, whatever the actual rates found in a particular study. This model can be simplified by setting the 'study' variable (S_i) to 0.

$$P = \exp (-13.50 + 0.137 X)$$

Jorm *et al.* termed this formula the **baseline model**. It is similar to Preston's and may be thought of as the average exponential curve derived from all studies. The study variable, S_i, has the effect of moving the exponential curve above or below this baseline model. Figure 4.1 shows the baseline model, as well as the statistical model's account of data from Campbell *et al.*'s (1983) New Zealand study and Hasegawa *et al.*'s (1986) Japanese study. Although the prevalence rates are much higher in the New Zealand study, the rise in prevalence with age is

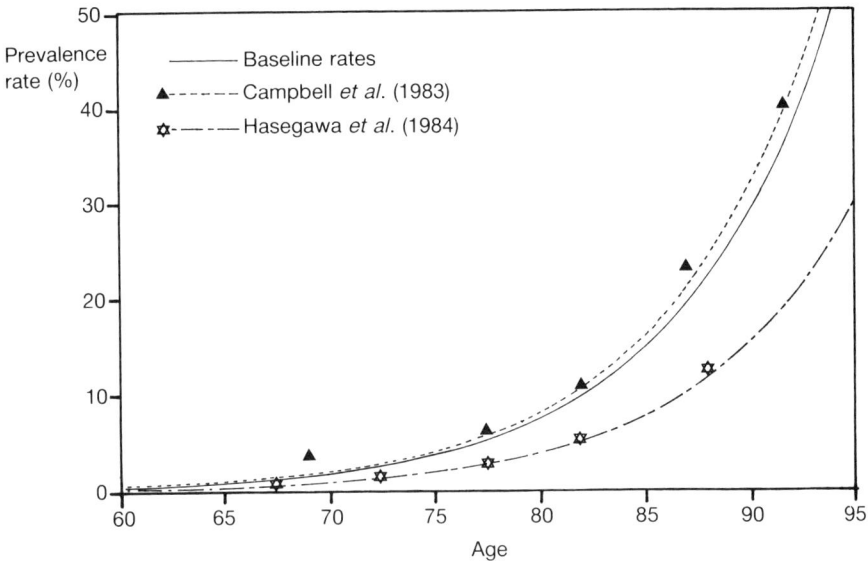

Figure 4.1 Age-specific prevalence rates according to the baseline model and selected studies. From Jorm *et al.* (1987).

exponential in both cases. The curve for the New Zealand data is very close to the average for all studies, leading to the result that Preston's formula (derived solely from the New Zealand data) yields rates very similar to those of the baseline model. The baseline model gives rates for specific ages, but rates for five-year age intervals can be derived by substituting an estimated median age for each interval. This procedure results in the prevalence rates shown in Table 4.5. Note that these rates apply to both males and females. Although some individual studies showed sex differences, these were not consistent from study to study, so that there was no overall sex difference in age-adjusted rates.

Table 4.5 Age-specific prevalence rates (%) derived from Jorm *et al.*'s (1987) baseline model

Age group	Median age	Prevalence rate
60–64	62.5	0.7
65–69	67.5	1.4
70–74	72.5	2.8
75–79	77.5	5.6
80–84	82.0	10.5
85–89	87.0	20.8
90–95	91.5	38.6

The prevalence rates derived from the baseline model should not be regarded as *the* rates for dementia. Rather, the conclusion from Jorm *et al.*'s (1987) analysis is that there is no simple answer to the question 'what is the prevalence of dementia?' The answer varies depending on the methods adopted for answering the question. Given a particular diagnostic instrument, diagnostic criteria and sampling methodology, an answer is possible. This conclusion has important implications for future prevalence studies. If there is to be a cumulation of knowledge about prevalence and a direct comparison of studies across different populations, then greater standardization of methodology is required. For researchers interested in estimating prevalence in a particular population for administrative purposes, the definition of dementia needs to be linked to the requirements of particular services. For example, if the allocation of resources to nursing home and hospital beds is the issue, then the degree of impairment for defining dementia could be linked to these needs. If it is accepted that the prevalence of dementia doubles with every 5.1 years of age, it is not necessary to estimate prevalence at all ages. If prevalence is estimated accurately for one particular age group (e.g. 70–75 year olds), the results can be used to extrapolate to other age groups in the population.

4.3 POPULATION DIFFERENCES IN PREVALENCE OF DEMENTIA

Prevalence studies are potentially useful for making comparisons between different populations. However, as discussed previously, methodological differences between studies make direct comparisons extremely difficult. Nevertheless, direct comparisons of prevalence are possible for sub-populations within a single study (e.g. sex or race differences) or between different populations which have been studied using a standard methodology. In this section, evidence on population differences in the dementia syndrome is reviewed, while evidence on specific dementing diseases is covered later in the chapter.

4.3.1 Sex differences

Jorm *et al.* (1987) examined sex differences in their statistical analyses of prevalence studies. There were 18 studies which gave separate male and female prevalence rates for those aged 65+, but the difference between the sexes was not significant. When 15 studies giving age-specific rates were examined, there was again no significant difference in rates. Although two of these studies did find a significant sex difference, they were in conflicting directions. We can safely conclude, therefore, that there is no overall sex difference in prevalence of the dementia syndrome.

4.3.2 Race differences

Race provides another area where within-study comparisons are possible. However, there are very few studies which have sufficient numbers of two races for prevalence differences to be studied reliably. Those studies that do exist are all from the United States. Weissman *et al.* (1985) and Kramer *et al.* (1985) have reported on race differences in cognitive impairment, which was defined by a low score on the Mini-Mental State Examination. Both studies found a higher prevalence of cognitive impairment amongst Blacks compared to Whites. Similarly, Gurland *et al.* (1983) found that Blacks had higher average scores than Whites on Rational Scale of Dementia which is essentially a cognitive screening test derived from a longer interview. However, cognitive impairment may result from pre-existing low cognitive ability as well as from dementia. From these studies, we cannot tell which is responsible. The only study to look specifically at dementia prevalence in Blacks and Whites was carried out by Schoenberg *et al.* (1985) in Southern USA. Consistent with the reports of higher prevalence of cognitive impairment in Blacks, Schoenberg *et al.* found a higher prevalence of dementia. Even so, the possible effect which premorbid race differences in cognitive ability could have on dementia diagnoses must be considered.

4.3.3 Differences between communities

Prevalence studies using standard methodologies in different communities are all too rare. The only systematic cross-national prevalence study is the US/UK study of Gurland *et al.* (1983). The study examined dementia prevalence in the elderly of New York and London. Copeland *et al.* (1987a) reported that prevalence was higher in New York than London, even though a computerized diagnostic algorithm (AGECAT) was used in conjunction with standard diagnostic interviews (GMS in London and CARE in New York). This difference was found to hold for both sexes and with all age groups from 65–69 up to 90+. No explanation could be found for the difference and it was hypothesized that an environmental factor could be responsible. Some other prevalence studies have used methodologies comparable to the US/UK study and so the rates can also be directly compared. Copeland *et al.* (1987b) found that the prevalence in Liverpool was closer to that in London than New York. However Kay *et al.* (1985) compared their results from Hobart, Australia, to the New York and London data, but found that Hobart had a higher rate like New York. Based on the limited evidence to date, there appears to be considerable scope for exploring cross-national differences in prevalence.

4.4 PROJECTED INCREASES IN PREVALENCE

One of the principal uses of prevalence studies is to assess service needs for dementia sufferers, not only in the present but also in the future. The world-wide experience of an increasingly ageing population has provoked considerable interest in assessing the effects of this trend on dementia prevalence. As a population ages, not only do the relative numbers of the elderly increase, but the very elderly become a larger proportion of the total elderly. An implication of this shift in the age distribution of the population is that any chronic diseases which are more prominent in the elderly will increase in prevalence.

There have been a number of attempts throughout the world to project increases in dementia cases. All such attempts have involved taking some age-specific prevalence rates and applying these to projections of population size in different age groups. This method assumes, of course, that there is no change in incidence or survival over the period of the projections. It simply examines the effects of a changing age structure on prevalence. Such an approach has been used by Kramer (1983) for the USA, by Ineichen (1987) for Britain, by Henderson (1983) for Australia and New Zealand, and by Rocca and Amaducci (1984) for a number of developed countries. The limitation of this method is that results may vary considerably depending on the particular age-specific prevalence rates that are used. For example, Jorm and Korten (1988) have reviewed quite different dementia projections for Australia which have resulted because of varying selection of published prevalence rates. If it is accepted that prevalence rates are dependent on the methodology used to determine them and that there is consequently no single set of 'true' rates, then there would appear to be no solution to the problem. There would always be a variety of legitimate projections, depending on the prevalence rates chosen. However, Jorm and Korten (1988) have pointed out that a resolution is possible if relative increases in prevalence are projected instead of absolute numbers of cases. They proposed a method based on Jorm *et al.*'s (1987) statistical model of prevalence: $P_i = \exp (S_i - 13.50 + 0.137\ X)$. If this model is used to make prevalence estimates for some base year (say 1984) and then projections to some later year (say 2000), the actual numbers estimated will depend on the value of the study variable (S_i) which is chosen. However, if the future prevalence is divided by the base-year prevalence, the percentage increase is the same whatever the value of S_i chosen. As an example, Jorm and Korten (1988) estimated dementia prevalence in Australia for 1984 and 1988, by setting S_i to 0. This gave figures of 87 170 and 100 290 cases. If, by contrast, the value of S_i had been set to -0.64 (a value derived from the study of Hasegawa *et al.* (1986)) then the numbers would be 45 980 for 1984 and 53 030 for 1988. However, in both cases, the increase from 1984 to 1988 is 15%. Because the same

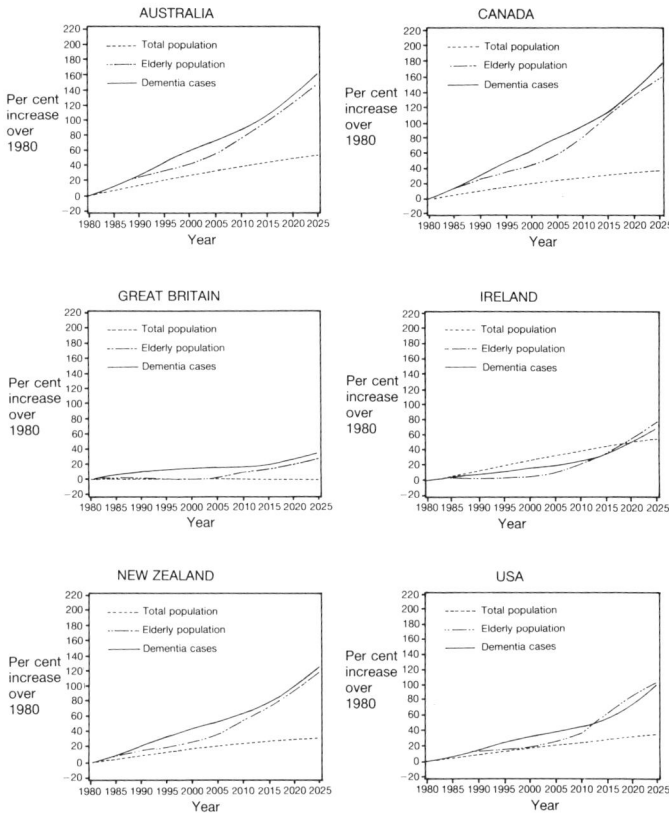

Figure 4.2 Projections of increases in dementia cases for six English-speaking countries. Adapted from Jorm *et al.* (1988b).

percentage increase in cases always results, it is simplest to set S_i to 0 and use the equation: $P = \exp(-13.50 + 0.137\, X)$.

This method of making projections has been applied to 29 developed countries using United Nations population projections (Jorm *et al.*, 1988b). These projections use 1980 as the base year and project up to 2025. Figure 4.2 shows the projections for six English-speaking countries. The actual percentage increases for all 29 countries are given in tabular form in Appendix C. While there is a general world-wide trend towards an ageing population, the projections for the developed countries show some striking differences. Some countries are expected to have a rapidly ageing population, but with dementia cases increasing at an even more rapid rate (e.g. Australia, Canada, Japan, New Zealand). In others, dementia cases are expected to grow at a slower rate, but still exceed the growth of the elderly as a total group (e.g. Great Britain, Sweden).

These latter countries are ones which already have relatively aged populations. The projections for France and East Germany are most unusual, because in these countries the elderly are growing at a faster rate than dementia cases – there is even expected to be some decrease in case numbers in the short term. Ireland also presents an unusual pattern: the increase in total population is expected to be greater than the increase in both the elderly and dementia cases. The more typical pattern of an ageing population will not occur there until the early decades of the next century.

All projections are necessarily uncertain. However, projections of the elderly population are less so than projections of the young, because the elderly of the future have already been born and can be counted. Only assumptions of future mortality need to be made in projecting the elderly population. To extend projections of the elderly to yield projections of dementia prevalence, we need to go further and assume that age-specific rates remain constant. If the incidence or survival of dementia cases were to change, then the projections would be affected in unknown ways. While future changes in incidence or survival are unknowable, there has been some investigation of past changes. In a population study in southern Sweden, Rorsman *et al.* (1985a, 1986) found no changes in incidence or survival over a 25-year period. Similarly, Kokmen *et al.* (1988) found no changes in incidence over a 15-year period in a US community.

4.5 PREVALENCE OF DEMENTING DISEASES

Although there are numerous studies of dementia prevalence, only a minority of these have attempted a clinical diagnosis of specific dementing diseases. The most important dementing diseases in the elderly are Alzheimer's disease, vascular dementia and mixed Alzheimer–vascular dementia. As discussed in Chapters 1 and 2, the clinical diagnosis of these diseases is difficult in the best of circumstances, but particularly so in the context of a field study. As criteria for clinical diagnosis have become more stringent, the difficulties for the field researcher have likewise increased. In the past, the practical demands of clinical diagnosis were less, but accuracy of diagnosis would have suffered as a consequence. For this reason, the results of earlier prevalence studies must be interpreted with caution. Even the terminology has changed considerably over the years. What we would today call clinically-diagnosed Alzheimer's disease might be called senile dementia, primary degenerative dementia, senile brain syndrome, or senile dementia of the Alzheimer type. Similarly, vascular dementia has been variously referred to as arteriosclerotic dementia, psychosis with cerebral arteriosclerosis and multi-infarct dementia. In reviewing the relevant literature, we are forced to assume that these terms refer to approximately equivalent diagnostic categories.

Because of the diagnostic uncertainty involved with prevalence studies, it is instructive to compare their results with clinic-based and neuro-pathological studies. There are a number of clinic-based studies which report on the prevalence of various diseases amongst cases seen at specialist dementia clinics. These studies suffer from the problem that only a biased group of dementia cases may be seen in such clinics. The advantage over community-based prevalence studies is, however, that much more thorough diagnostic procedures can be carried out on cases who have sought assistance from a clinic. Another source of evidence about the relative prevalence of specific dementing diseases comes from neuropathological studies. These studies involve additional bias in that only a small minority of diagnosed dementia cases will come to autopsy and these may well be unrepresentative. However, combined neuro-pathological and clinical investigation provides certain diagnosis and eliminates error in this area. In summary, we have a trade-off between representativeness of samples and accuracy of diagnosis. Field studies of prevalence provide the greatest representativeness but least accuracy, while neuropathological studies provide diagnostic accuracy but at the expense of representativeness. Clinic-based studies are somewhere in between. In practice, any findings which are confirmed in all types of studies will inspire greater confidence. Below we examine the evidence on the distribution of the major dementing diseases as a function of four factors: age, sex, region and race.

4.5.1 Age differences

Jorm *et al.* (1987) showed that dementia prevalence rises exponentially with age across studies, although the rates actually reported varied from study to study. Similar findings emerged when they analysed seven studies giving separate age-specific rates for Alzheimer's disease and vascular dementia. One study could not be fitted well by an exponential model, but this appeared to be due to oddities in its sampling method-ology. The others were well described by a model showing that Alzheimer's disease rates double with every 4.5 years of age, while vascular dementia rates double with every 5.3 years. In other words, the rise with age was steeper for Alzheimer's disease. The exponential rise appears to continue at least to age 90, but beyond that little can be concluded because of the small number of extremely old subjects found in prevalence studies. If the exponential rise were to continue, then a point would be reached where everybody living long enough would have these dementing diseases. Although Jorm *et al.*'s analysis revealed that the underlying age trend across studies is exponential, there were differences between studies in the actual rates and in the relative importance of Alzheimer and vascular dementias.

Some other evidence on age differences comes from neuropathological studies of individuals dying at various ages. These studies tell us about prevalence at age of death. This may, of course, be different from the prevalence amongst people of the same age who are alive. Given that dementia is associated with reduced survival, individuals dying at a particular age will have a higher prevalence than those surviving. Nevertheless, the age trends involved are of considerable interest. Several studies have looked at the prevalence of senile plaques, neuro-fibrillary tangles or granulovacuolar degeneration at death. Since no clinical data were available on the presence or absence of dementia in these individuals, they are studies of Alzheimer brain changes rather than Alzheimer's disease *per se*. The general finding is that Alzheimer brain changes increase steeply with age at death. Table 4.6 shows data from a US study of 199 autopsied individuals by Miller *et al.* (1984). The age trend of having 'many plaques and many tangles' could roughly be described as exponential. Other studies show similar age trends up to age 90 or so (e.g. Stam *et al.*, 1986). Davies *et al.* (1988) found a similar age rise when they examined a series of brains for deposition of the A4 amyloid protein. This protein (also known as the β protein) is a major constituent of senile plaques. Prevalence of A4 was found to increase from 19% in the sixth decade to 79% in the ninth decade. Studies examining Alzheimer neuropathology over the age of 90, however, show a decline rather than a continued rise (Matsuyama and Nakamura, 1978; Peress *et al.*, 1978; Tomlinson and Kitchener, 1972). These findings can be interpreted as indicating that individuals who live to extreme old age are a survival elite who are less prone to Alzheimer's disease than the majority who die at earlier ages. However, caution is needed in interpreting data on prevalence at death. It could be, for example, that centenarians who are affected by Alzheimer's disease die early in the disease, generally of other causes, while affected individuals in their 80s are more likely to live the full course of the disease. Such a difference could easily produce a reduced prevalence of Alzheimer changes at death in the older age group, even if the incidence in those alive was higher in this group.

Table 4.6 Percentage of autopsied individuals with many plaques and many tangles. Adapted from Miller *et al.* (1984)

Age group	Per cent affected
<55	0
55–64	3
65–74	5
75–84	20
85+	45

4.5.2 Sex differences

Jorm *et al.*'s (1987) analysis of dementia prevalence studies showed no overall sex difference. However, a different finding emerged when studies of specific dementing diseases were analysed. Rates for Alzheimer's disease tended to be higher among females than males, whereas rates for vascular dementia tended to be higher for males. Table 4.7 shows their summary of data from 13 relevant studies. While the limitations of clinical diagnosis in field studies suggest caution in the interpretation of this sex difference, other evidence confirms its existence.

Table 4.7 Prevalence of Alzheimer's disease and vascular dementia by sex (rates are simple averages of reported rates in per cent). Adapted from Jorm *et al.* (1987)

Region	Number of studies	Alzheimer		Vascular	
		Males	Females	Males	Females
Japan	4	0.8	1.5	3.3	2.7
Russia	1	1.1	3.8	6.1	2.1
Scandinavia	3	1.6	2.2	1.0	1.4
Britain	3	3.0	4.9	4.4	2.7
USA	2	0.7	2.1	3.5	0.8

Neuropathological studies of dementia cases consistently show that females predominate amongst Alzheimer's disease cases (Tomlinson *et al.*, 1970; Birkett, 1972; Morimatsu *et al.*, 1975; Wilcock and Esiri, 1982; St Clair and Whalley, 1983; Nishihari and Ishii, 1986; Ojeda *et al.*, 1986; Wade *et al.*, 1987). Part of this effect is probably due to there being more females than males dying with dementing diseases generally; since females tend to live longer, they are more prone to die with any age-related disease. However, the same studies mostly show an excess of males amongst vascular dementia cases (Tomlinson *et al.*, 1970; Birkett, 1972; Morimatsu *et al.*, 1975; St Clair and Whalley, 1983; Nishihari and Ishii, 1986; Wade *et al.*, 1987).

In addition to these neuropathological studies of dementia cases, there are studies of Alzheimer neuropathology in large unselected autopsy samples. Skullerud (1985) in Norway found Alzheimer changes to be more common in women, while Stam *et al.* (1986) in the Netherlands found that senile plaques had both a higher prevalence and a sharper increase with age in women. However, other studies have failed to find a sex difference in Alzheimer neuropathology. In Miller *et al.*'s (1984) US study there was no sex difference in plaque and tangle frequency when age was controlled. Matsuyama and Nakamura (1978) similarly found no age-specific sex difference in plaque and tangle frequency in a Japanese autopsy series. Davies *et al.* (1988) in Australia, examined a series of elderly brains for A4 (or β) amyloid protein deposition and found no sex difference.

Other relevant evidence comes from studies of cerebrovascular disease incidence. Haberman *et al.* (1981) have reviewed these studies and concluded that there is a higher stroke incidence in males than females. This higher rate potentially explains the sex difference in prevalence of vascular dementia.

Clinic-based studies provide yet another potential source of information on sex differences, but, unfortunately, these generally fail to report data on the issue. An exception is a study by Thal *et al.* (1988) which, consistent with other evidence, reported an excess of females amongst Alzheimer cases and an excess of males amongst vascular cases.

4.5.3 Regional differences

Because of the varying methodologies of different studies, it is seldom possible to compare directly prevalence rates obtained from different regions. An exception is the study by Sulkava *et al.* (1988) on dementia prevalence for the whole of Finland. They used an identical case-ascertainment procedure in various parts of the country, but still found regional differences. The prevalence of Alzheimer's disease was significantly higher in the north and east of Finland compared to the rest of the country. However, the prevalence of vascular dementia did not differ significantly between regions. The reason for these regional differences is unknown.

While the absolute prevalence rates from different studies may not be comparable, the relative prevalence of Alzheimer's disease and vascular dementia can be usefully compared. It is generally believed that Alzheimer's disease is the most common dementing disease, but this may not be the case in all parts of the world. If the predominance of Alzheimer's disease is found in only some countries, then this might provide important clues to the aetiology of the major dementing diseases. There must be some environmental or genetic factor which accounts for such differences.

Table 4.8 shows the most common dementing diseases in prevalence studies carried out in various countries and regions. While Alzheimer's disease appears to be the most common in Western Europe and North America, vascular dementia is reported to predominate in Japan, Russia and China. It may be that regional effects are due to differences in diagnostic practice rather than to true differences in the relative prevalence of Alzheimer and vascular dementias. It is possible to look to clinic-

Table 4.8 Most common dementing diseases in prevalence studies from various countries and regions

Region	Studies showing Alzheimer's disease to be most common	Studies showing vascular dementia to be most common
Scandinavia	Åkesson (1969) Mölsä *et al.* (1982) Rorsman *et al.* (1986) Sulkava *et al.* (1985a)	Bollerup (1975)
Britain	Brayne and Calloway (1989) Broe *et al.* (1976) Gurland *et al.* (1983) Kay *et al.* (1964a) O'Connor *et al.* (1989c) Primrose (1962)	
North America	Evans *et al.* (1990) Gurland *et al.* (1983) Kokmen *et al.* (1989) Schoenberg *et al.* (1985)	Folstein *et al.* (1985)
Southern Europe	D'Alessandro *et al.* (1988) Lippi *et al.* (1989) Pinessi *et al.* (1984)	
Russia		Gawrilova (1984) Gawrilova *et al.* (1987) Sternberg and Gawrilowa (1978)
Japan		Hasegawa *et al.* (1983) Hasegawa *et al.* (1986) Kaneko (1975) Karasawa *et al.* (1982) Makiya (1978) Motohiro *et al.* (1985) Shibayama *et al.* (1986)
China		Chen (1987) Kuang and Zhao (1984) Li *et al.* (1989) Zhao (1986)

based and neuropathological studies for confirming evidence. Clinic-based studies uniformly show a preponderance of Alzheimer's disease. Most of these studies have been carried out in North America (Freemon, 1976; Hutton, 1981; Rabins, 1981; Maletta *et al.*, 1982; Cummings and

Benson, 1983; Larson *et al.*, 1985; Thal *et al.*, 1988) with others in Britain (Marsden and Harrison, 1972; Victoratos *et al.*, 1977), Australia (Smith and Kiloh, 1981) and Finland (Erkinjuntti *et al.*, 1987b). Unfortunately, there are no studies of this type in the countries where prevalence studies show higher rates of vascular dementia. The results of neuro-pathological studies are shown in Table 4.9. It can be seen that Alzheimer's disease predominates in Western Europe, North America, Russia and Australia. By contrast, the Japanese neuropathological studies show vascular dementia to be the most common. Unfortunately, there are as yet no neuropathological studies from China.

Given the consistency of results between community, clinic-based and neuropathological studies in Western Europe and North America, we can safely conclude that Alzheimer's disease is the most common cause of dementia in these regions. For Russia, by contrast, there is conflicting evidence, with prevalence studies showing vascular dementia to be more common and a neuropathological study showing Alzheimer's

Table 4.9 Most common dementing diseases in neuropathological studies from various countries and regions

Region	Studies showing Alzheimer's disease to be most common	Studies showing vascular dementia to be most common
Scandinavia	Gustafson and Nilsson (1982) Mölsä *et al.* (1985) Sourander and Sjögren (1970)	
Britain	St Clair and Whalley (1983) Tomlinson *et al.* (1970) Wilcock and Esiri (1982)	Homer *et al.* (1988)
North America	Boller *et al.* (1989) Kokmen *et al.* (1987) Müller and Schwartz (1978) Rosen *et al.* (1980) Wade *et al.* (1987)	Birkett (1972)
Central Europe	Jellinger (1976) Todorov *et al.* (1975)	
Russia	Shefer (1987)	
Australia	Ojeda *et al.* (1986)	
Japan	Morimatsu *et al.* (1975)	Matsushita and Ishii (1979) Nishihara and Ishii (1986) Tomonaga (1979)

disease to be more common. More recently, Shefer (1987) has carried out a neuropathological follow-up of dementia cases diagnosed by Russian psychiatrists and concluded that they substantially over-diagnose vascular dementia. Therefore, the results of the Russian prevalence studies are probably a diagnostic artefact. However, the results from the Japanese studies cannot be explained this way. Both prevalence and neuropathological studies fairly consistently show an excess of vascular dementia over Alzheimer's disease. In the only neuropathological study to give contrary findings (Morimatsu *et al.*, 1975), the excess of Alzheimer's disease was small and there was a large mixed dementia group. Why the Japanese show relatively more vascular dementia is unknown: their rate of Alzheimer's disease could be lower than for Caucasian peoples or their rate of vascular dementia higher. Because it is impossible to compare absolute prevalence rates across different studies, the two possibilities cannot be distinguished in the available data. A cross-national study using the same methodology in various countries is needed. However, there is some indirect evidence that an increased rate of vascular dementia in Japan is responsible for the difference. A cross-national study of stroke, using identical procedures in different countries, found particularly high rates in Japan (Aho *et al.*, 1980). As for China, the high relative prevalence of vascular dementia shown in prevalence studies must await other confirming evidence.

Given that regional differences appear to exist, there is a need for data on the prevalence of dementing diseases in other parts of the world. There is no information available on their prevalence in Africa, Latin America or much of Asia. If further regional differences can be found, they may give valuable clues to the aetiology of Alzheimer or vascular dementias.

4.5.4 Race differences

As discussed previously, rarely do prevalence studies contain sufficient numbers of two races for differences in prevalence to be studied. Rarer still are studies which also involve clinical diagnosis of specific dementing diseases. Only one study to date has addressed this issue. Schoenberg *et al.* (1985) studied a population in the Southern USA where Blacks and Whites live in roughly equal numbers. They were able to carry out a clinical diagnosis of Alzheimer's disease and found age-adjusted rates to be somewhat higher in Blacks. Such a difference may reflect either increased incidence or survival amongst Blacks. However, increased survival was thought to be unlikely with this group, so a true racial difference in incidence could be involved.

Only one neuropathological study has looked at race differences. Miller *et al.* (1984) found that Blacks were somewhat more likely than

Whites to have many plaques and tangles at death. Although this difference was not statistically significant, Miller *et al.* concluded that 'a slight difference could exist in the larger population' (p. 337).

4.6 THE FUTURE OF PREVALENCE STUDIES

Prevalence has been, and continues to be, a major focus of research in the epidemiology of dementing diseases. Most of the studies carried out to date have concerned single populations in which the crude prevalence rates are estimated for global dementia. However, there would seem little point in any further studies of this type. Because of the idiosyncratic methodologies of such studies, it is impossible to compare directly results across populations. Of more value are studies in different populations using a standard methodology. There is also little use in crude prevalence rates for ages 60+ or 65+. In a situation where the age structure of the world's populations is rapidly changing, such crude prevalence estimates soon become dated. Finally, there is a need for information on the prevalence of specific dementing diseases diagnosed using acceptable criteria. In the context of a field study, diagnosis of specific diseases may prove impossible to do well until an accurate biological test for Alzheimer's disease is developed. Nevertheless, the feasibility of methods of clinical diagnosis needs exploration.

5   Incidence

While differences between populations in prevalence are of considerable interest, they are ambiguous because such effects could reflect differences in either incidence or survival. Despite their greater theoretical importance, incidence studies are far less numerous than prevalence studies. The reason is that incidence studies require longitudinal observation to ascertain new onsets of dementing diseases. As well, because the annual rate of onsets is generally small, incidence studies require either large sample sizes or long follow-ups to estimate rates reliably. Table 5.1 lists the incidence studies carried out to date on general population samples using acceptable case ascertainment procedures. There are other studies which give incidence date, but are limited because of their case ascertainment or sampling procedure. Sayetta (1986) has given incidence data from a sample of volunteer American men, while

Table 5.1   Studies of the incidence of Alzheimer's disease and related disorders

Author(s)	Year	Country	Age-specific rates	Specific dementing disorders
Åkesson	1969	Sweden	Yes	Yes
Bergmann et al.	1971	Britain	No	Yes
Bickel and Cooper	1989	Germany	Yes	No
Gurland et al.	1983	Britain and USA	No	No
Hagnell et al.	1983	Sweden	Yes	Yes
Helgason; Magnusson and Helgason	1973; 1981	Iceland	Yes	No
Maule et al.	1984	Britain	No	No
Mölsä et al.	1982	Finland	Yes	Yes
Nielsen et al.	1981	Denmark	Yes	No
Nilsson	1984	Sweden	Yes	Yes
Schoenberg et al.	1987	USA	Yes	Yes
Treves et al.	1986	Israel	Yes (pre-senile only)	Yes

incidence data based on hospitalization or contact with psychiatric services has been reported by Larsson *et al.* (1963), Adelstein *et al.* (1968), Reimann and Häfner (1972), Wing and Hailey (1972), Helgason (1977) and Hofman (1987).

Reviewing incidence studies involves the same problem as reviewing prevalence studies, i.e. the widely differing methodologies of the studies makes direct comparison of results difficult. For this reason, clear conclusions about group differences in incidence can generally only be drawn by making comparisons of subgroups within a population. Another limitation facing the reviewer is that the studies in Table 5.1 cover a limited area of the world. With the exception of two studies from the United States and one from Israel, all come from north-western Europe. Given this limited geographical and ethnic spread, any conclusions about the incidence of dementing disorders may not be generalizable to other populations. While keeping these limitations in mind, this chapter reviews the effects on incidence of age, sex, ethnicity, region and historical period.

5.1 AGE DIFFERENCES

As discussed in the previous chapter, the prevalence of dementia rises exponentially with age, at least up to age 90. Given that age differences in survival are unlikely to produce such a trend, we might expect a similar sort of age rise in incidence. Figure 5.1 summarizes the available data on the issue. Figure 5.1(a) gives the results from studies which have reported only on the dementia syndrome while (b) and (c) are based on studies giving incidence of specific dementing diseases. A striking feature of these results is the substantial differences in incidence among the studies. To some extent, these differences are associated with the level of severity being assessed, with studies of moderate-to-severe dementia having higher rates than those of severe dementia only. However, there are notable exceptions. For example the study by Mölsä *et al.* (1982) which claims to ascertain 'moderate to severe' dementia has lower rates than Nilsson's (1984) study of 'severe dementia'. Ignoring these differences in the absolute values of incidence and focusing on the underlying age trends, it can be seen that incidence rises substantially with age. Generally speaking, the incidence rates between the ages of 60 and 90 involve an upward swing suggestive of an exponential rise. There are, as well, studies of the incidence of cognitive impairment which show a similar age trend (Eaton *et al.*, 1989; Jagger *et al.*, 1989).

5.1.1 Incidence in the very old

While the studies graphed in Figure 5.1 show an increase in incidence with age, Mortimer *et al.* (1981) have speculated that incidence may

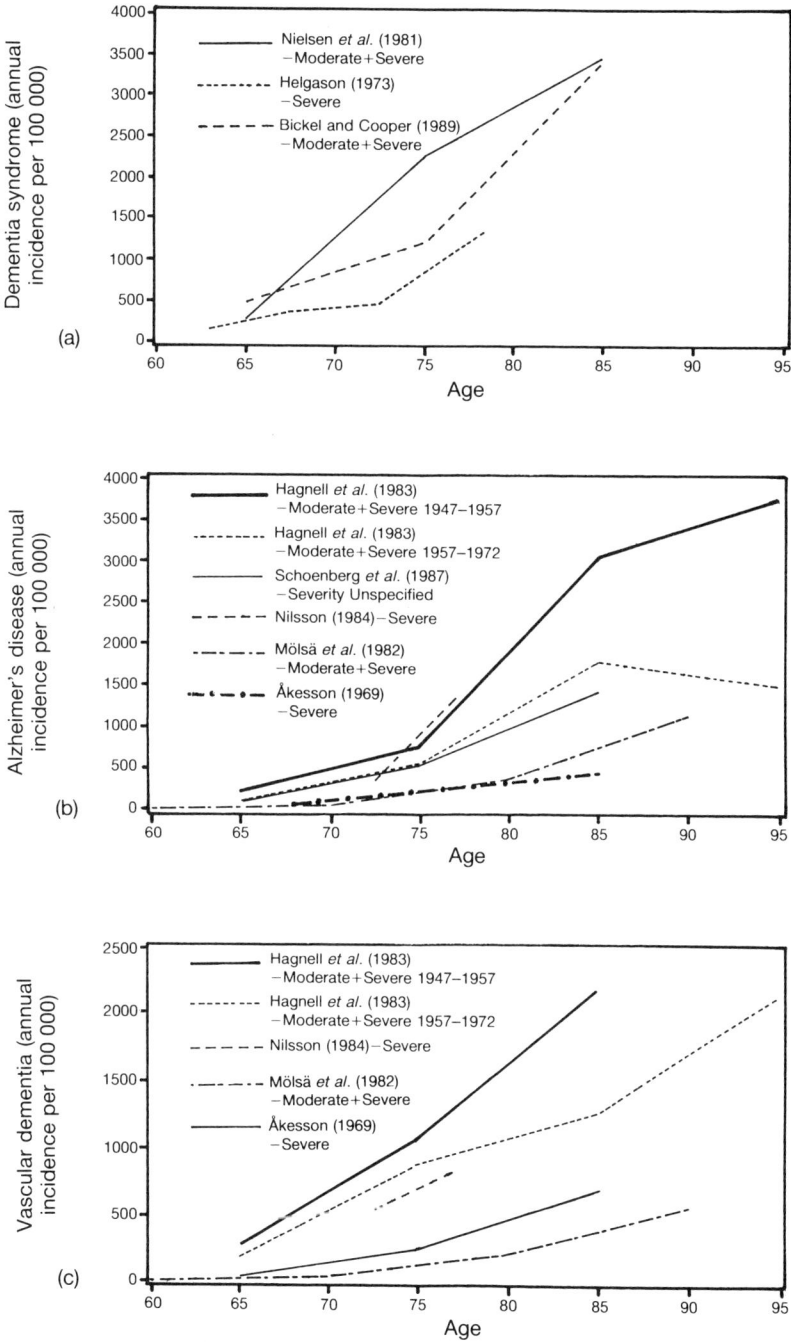

Figure 5.1 Age-specific incidence rates for the dementia syndrome and for specific dementing diseases.

begin to level off in the very old. This view is based on data from Larsson *et al.* (1963) on psychiatric hospital admissions. This study found a levelling off at around 75 years of age. However, psychiatric admissions measure only treated incidence and provide a biased estimate of total incidence. Of the studies shown in Figure 5.1, only the one by Hagnell *et al.* (1983) showed any levelling off in the very old. In that study, the levelling occurred only for Alzheimer's disease over the age of 85. However, the number of subjects on which incidence estimates are based inevitably becomes very small when dealing with this age group. The results may reflect unreliability in the data rather than a true levelling. The only other study to report on incidence past 85 years is that of Mölsä *et al.* (1982) and they found a continued rise.

Mortimer *et al.* (1981) have cited a number of neuropathological studies of Alzheimer brain changes as supporting the incidence data of Larsson *et al.* (1963). These studies found a levelling, or even decline, in Alzheimer neuropathology in individuals dying over the age of 90. However, as pointed out in the previous chapter, these are studies of prevalence at death rather than incidence, and the results could reflect age differences in survival of Alzheimer's cases. If older cases were to die earlier in the disease, then there might be a decline in the prevalence of Alzheimer neuropathology at death.

5.1.2 Lifetime risk of Alzheimer's disease

For practical purposes, what happens to incidence over age 90 is of little interest because so few individuals survive past this age. However, it is of great theoretical importance because it addresses the issue of whether everyone would develop Alzheimer's disease if they lived long enough. If Alzheimer's disease was inevitable given a sufficiently long lifespan, then it might be better viewed as a normal part of ageing rather than a disease state. If, on the other hand, a substantial proportion of the population would never develop Alzheimer's disease, then it is more properly seen as a disease superimposed on ageing. In considering whether Alzheimer's disease is inevitable, we need to consider the lifetime risk of the disorder and its relationship to incidence rates. The lifetime risk is the chance of developing a disease for individuals who live up to a certain age. This risk can be calculated from age-specific incidence rates, as explained in Chapter 3. If Alzheimer's disease was inevitable, then the lifetime risk would asymptote at 100% by some extreme age. On the other hand, if the disease was caused by some genetic factor or environmental exposure confined to a proportion of the population, the lifetime risk would level off at less than 100%. For example, Chase *et al.* (1983) have hypothesized that an autosomal dominant gene is involved in Alzheimer's disease. This theory predicts

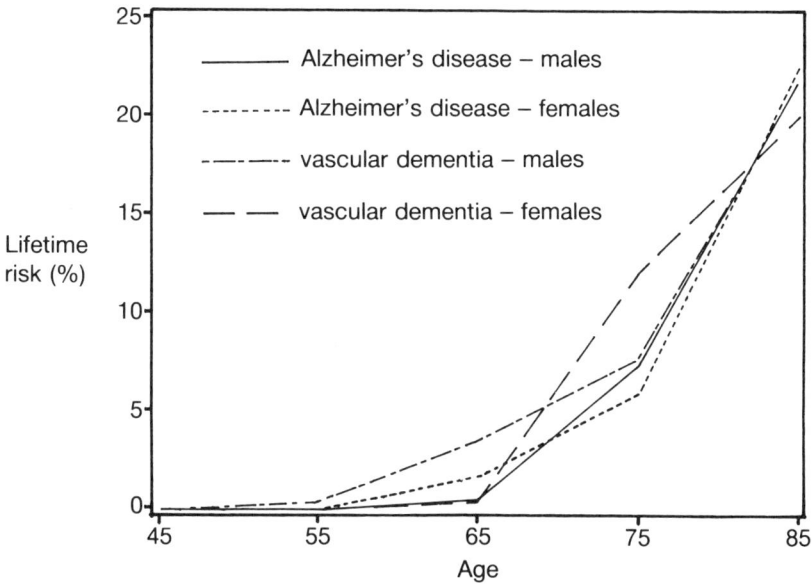

Figure 5.2 Lifetime risk for dementing diseases (moderate–severe) according to data from the Lundby study, 1957–1972.

that lifetime risk will level off at around 50% for first-degree relatives of sufferers, and at a rate much lower than this in the rest of the population. Any studies giving age-specific incidence data can be used for calculating lifetime risk. However, of these studies, the Lundby study (Hagnell *et al.*, 1983) provides the most interesting data because of the broad age range it encompassed and its low threshold for ascertaining cases. Data from this study have been used to calculate lifetime risk up to age 89 (Hagnell *et al.*, 1983) and this is shown graphically in Figure 5.2. It can be seen that the risk up to this age is far less than 100%, yet at the same time, there is no hint of a levelling off in the risk.

While it might seem that a decline in incidence in extreme old age would imply that the lifetime risk levels off at less than 100%, this is not necessarily so. Figure 5.3 shows some theoretical possibilities for incidence and lifetime risk. In Figure 5.3, the incidence continues rising into extreme old age. Such a rise implies that, at any extreme age, only a small proportion of survivors would be unaffected and these would have a very high probability of themselves becoming demented in the coming year. This incidence function has an associated lifetime risk curve where risk rises steeply with age and then begins to level off just before the asymptote of 100%. However, incidence does not have to

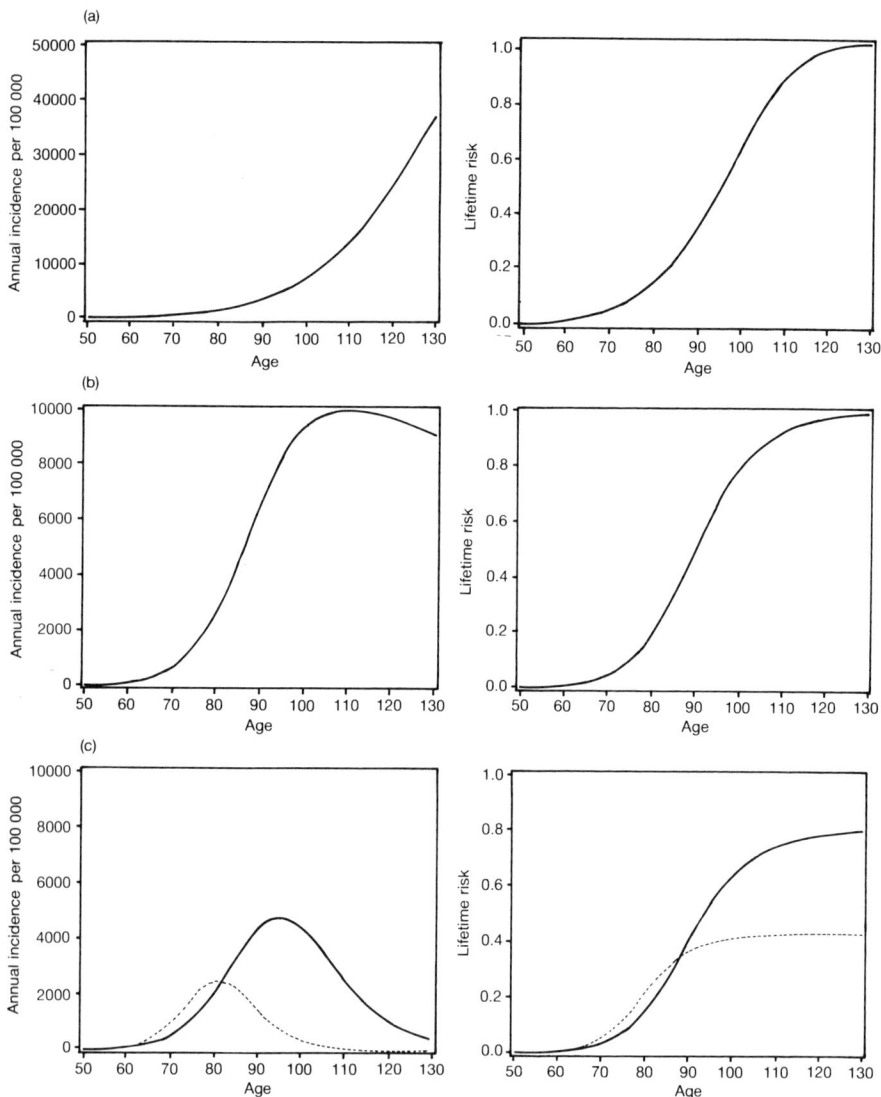

Figure 5.3 Some theoretical possibilities for incidence and lifetime risk.

continue rising for lifetime risk to approach 100%. Figure 5.3(b) shows a situation where incidence rises to a peak and then declines; nevertheless, the associated lifetime risk curve continues to rise. Figure 5.3(c) shows two other examples where there is a rise and fall in incidence, but with the overall rates being lower. In both these examples, the lifetime risk levels off at something less than 100%. Such situations might arise if a specific gene was responsible, but varied in its age of expression according to the presence or absence of various other factors. The rate at which risk levelled off would reflect the type of gene involved (dominant or recessive, sex-linked or autosomal) and its frequency in the population. An asymptote of less than 100% would establish that a pathological process, distinct from normal ageing, was involved.

As theoretically interesting as these possibilities are, they are extremely difficult to test empirically because of the small number of people surviving to the ages where a decline in incidence could plausibly occur. Such a study would require a substantial number of people aged over 100 and this sample could not be assembled except by large-scale international co-operative effort. If the decline was hypothesized to occur at age 110 or over, then such a study would be impossible since the record lifespan for most developed countries is around this age.

5.2 SEX DIFFERENCES

In Chapter 4 it was reported that there is no overall sex difference in prevalence of dementia across studies. The incidence studies, however, yield rather inconsistent results, with some showing no sex difference (Helgason, 1973; Hagnell *et al.*, 1981; Schoenberg *et al.*, 1987), others showing a higher incidence in females (Åkesson, 1969; Mölsä *et al.*, 1982), and one showing a higher rate in males (Nilsson, 1984). These inconsistencies are puzzling and perhaps relate to differences in case ascertainment procedures. They cannot be due to regional differences, since even studies carried out on the west coast of Sweden show apparently conflicting results (Åkesson, 1969; Nilsson, 1984).

With specific dementing diseases, prevalence rates for Alzheimer's disease tend to be higher for females, while prevalence rates for vascular dementia tend to be higher for males. Incidence studies show similar trends, but they are not clear-cut. Of the six studies reporting on sex differences in Alzheimer's disease, three show females to have higher incidence (Åkesson, 1969; Mölsä *et al.*, 1982; Hagnell *et al.*, 1983), two show no difference (Treves *et al.*, 1986; Schoenberg *et al.*, 1987), and one shows a higher male incidence (Nilsson, 1984). Only four studies report on sex differences in vascular dementia. Two of these show a higher male rate (Hagnell *et al.*, 1983; Nilsson, 1984), one shows no sex difference (Åkesson, 1969) and the other shows a weak trend for a higher female rate (Mölsä *et al.*, 1982). The more consistent sex differences found in prevalence studies may, of course, reflect survival differences. The evidence on this issue is considered in the next chapter.

5.3 ETHNIC DIFFERENCES

Only one incidence study has examined ethnic differences within a community. Treves *et al.* (1986) estimated the incidence of Alzheimer's disease up to 60 years of age in Israel, using records of all patients discharged from hospitals. They found the incidence in Jews of European or American origin to be double that in Jews of African or Asian origin. While these results suggest a true ethnic difference in incidence, differential use of hospital services is an alternative explanation. Although hospital services are freely available in Israel, Jews born in Africa or Asia might be more likely to care for relatives at home. If this ethnic difference turns out to be real, it merits further investigation of genetic or environmental factors which might produce it.

Black/White differences in incidence in the USA provide another fruitful area for investigation. Schoenberg *et al.* (1987) have observed a somewhat higher prevalence of Alzheimer's disease in Blacks and this seems unlikely to be due to their longer survival. Consequently, a race difference in incidence is implicated.

5.4 REGIONAL DIFFERENCES

The only study to report on regional differences in incidence using a standard methodology in both regions is the US/UK Cross-National Project (Gurland *et al.*, 1983). As reported in the previous chapter, this study found a higher prevalence of dementia in New York than London. When the samples were followed up one year later, the incidence of new cases was also found to be higher in New York (2.4%) than in London (0.4%). This difference remains unexplained.

While incidence rates from different studies cannot be directly compared, the relative incidence of Alzheimer's disease and vascular dementia can be legitimately examined. Prevalence studies from Western Europe

Table 5.2   Most common dementing diseases in incidence studies from various countries

Study	Country	Most common dementing disease
Åkesson (1969)	Sweden	Vascular dementia
Bergmann *et al.* (1971)	Britain	Alzheimer's disease
Hagnell *et al.* (1983)	Sweden	Little difference between Alzheimer's and vascular dementias
Mölsä *et al.* (1982)	Finland	Alzheimer's disease
Nilsson (1984)	Sweden	Alzheimer's disease
Schoenberg *et al.* (1987)	USA	Alzheimer's disease

and North America tend to show Alzheimer's disease as the most prevalent dementia, whereas in Japan, Russia and China, vascular dementia is claimed to be more prevalent. Incidence studies are unfortunately available from only a limited part of the world; in particular, there are none from countries where a greater prevalence of vascular dementia is claimed. However, what evidence is available tends to support the view that Alzheimer's disease is the form of dementia with the highest incidence in north-western Europe and North America. Table 5.2 summarizes the results of these studies.

5.5 HISTORICAL PERIOD DIFFERENCES

The epidemiological study of dementing diseases is a relatively recent activity, so little information is available on whether incidence has changed over time. A notable exception is the Lundby study. This study began in 1947 when Essen-Möller *et al.* (1956) investigated psychiatric morbidity in a complete community of southern Sweden. This cohort was followed up in 1957 and 1972 by Hagnell and his colleagues. In addition, any newcomers to the area in 1957 were also added to the study. Thus, the original cohort was followed over a period of 25 years and the newcomers over a period of 15 years. Hagnell *et al.* (1981) reported that the age-specific incidence of dementia had decreased in the original Lundby cohort between 1947 and 1957 and 1957 and 1972. Later, incidence rates were calculated separately for clinically-diagnosed Alzheimer's disease and vascular dementia and both were found to decrease from the first to the second period. However, when Rorsman *et al.* (1986) included the newcomers in the incidence calculation, no significant difference was found between the two time periods for either dementing disease. Even if the Lundby data had shown a statistically reliable change in incidence, this could be questioned on methodological grounds. The original diagnosis in 1947 was carried out by Essen-Möller and colleagues, while the fieldwork was done by Hagnell in 1957 and Hagnell and Öjesjö in 1972. Although the training of these clinicians may have been similar, any difference between them in the cut-off for diagnosing dementia would have affected the incidence rates. Thus, if Essen-Möller and colleagues had a higher threshold for detecting cases in 1947 than Hagnell in 1957 and 1972, the incidence rate would be artifactually higher in the second time period. An adequate assessment of historical changes in incidence requires the use of highly standardized diagnostic procedures.

The only other attempt to assess historical changes in incidence was carried out by Kokmen *et al.* (1988) in the United States. They studied the medical records of the population of Rochester, Minnesota, over the period 1960–1974. The incidence of dementia ascertained from the records did not change over this period. However, with the method of case ascertainment used, cases of dementia which did not come to medical attention were excluded.

5.6 THE FUTURE OF INCIDENCE STUDIES

Methodological factors can greatly influence the rates obtained in incidence studies, just as they can in prevalence studies. Because of the confounding of true differences in incidence with methodological effects, it is not possible directly to compare rates derived from different studies. It is therefore useless to try to estimate *the* incidence of dementing diseases. Such estimates only have meaning in relation to other estimates obtained with a comparable methodology. Thus, future incidence studies need to focus on differences between subgroups within a population (e.g. age, sex or ethnic differences) or else compare incidence in different populations using a standard methodology.

While most incidence studies have examined age-specific incidence, some have only estimated crude incidence for the elderly as a group. Because of the changing age-structure of the elderly population, and the differences in age structure between populations, such estimates are of limited use as they will be affected by the relative weight of the very elderly in the total elderly population. Of great interest is the incidence of dementing diseases in extreme old age, particularly whether incidence continues to rise or decline in this age group. The answer may influence whether we regard disorders like Alzheimer's disease as pathological states or as a normal part of human ageing.

6 *Survival and mortality*

The study of survival is epidemiologically important because, along with the incidence rate, it is a determinant of the prevalence of a disease. The practical use of studying survival is in health services planning. It will be a factor in the burden on family care-givers, the demand for medical and welfare services and the turnover of long-term care beds.

Survival must be measured from some meaningful point in time. There are several possible time-points which can be used.

1. *Point of disease onset.* This time-point is the most useful for theoretical purposes, because, in combination with incidence, duration from onset determines the prevalence of a disease. The point at which any disease starts is difficult to specify, but the uncertainties are even greater with diseases like Alzheimer's which have an insidious onset. In studies which attempt this difficult task, two methods are possible: prospective and retrospective dating. Prospective dating involves following a sample longitudinally to detect any new cases. Onsets can then be dated as occurring between the points of longitudinal observation. The alternative is to date onset retrospectively by questioning informants about the timing of certain critical behavioural changes. This method will suffer not only from the problem of detecting an onset point with an insidious disease, but also from the memory limitations of the informants. Usually, retrospective dating of onset is carried out with formally diagnosed cases. Those cases that die before recognition, or are not formally recognized, will be excluded from the sample and so bias the results.

2. *Point of diagnosis.* Although survival from point of diagnosis is easily determined, it is theoretically less important than survival from onset. The exception is in epidemiological research using the case register method. In such research, incidence, prevalence and survival are all defined in terms of recognition of cases by services. As well, survival from diagnosis is of practical interest in guiding family members as to the future demands for care which they will face. However, the point at which a dementing disease is formally recognized may well be influenced by the nature of a community's health-care system. Recognition may be earlier in some than others, thus affecting survival figures. For this reason, figures on survival from

diagnosis may not be easily generalized from one community to another.

3. *Point of admission to long-term care.* Survival from admission to long-term care is easily determined from institutional records and, for this reason, is the most common type of survival studied. However, it is of little theoretical importance, being influenced by the admission policy of the particular institution studied. Some institutions may take more severe cases then others which will, of course, influence duration of survival. There may also be various socio-demographic biases in admission, e.g. cases of a particular sex, marital status or age group may be more likely to be admitted. The main use of this measure of survival is for determining institutional service needs.

While the most useful survival studies are those dating onset from longitudinal observations, such studies are rare. For this reason, studies of survival from diagnosis or admission often provide the only information available. Where all three types of survival measures provide consistent results, we can have greater confidence in any conclusions. We begin by examining the most basic question about survival in Alzheimer's disease and related disorders – whether these diseases shorten the lives of sufferers. The influence of various other variables on survival in dementing diseases is then examined.

6.1 REDUCTION IN SURVIVAL

In 1976, Katzman published an editorial on 'The prevalence and malignancy of Alzheimer disease' in which he argued that both Alzheimer and vascular dementias produced a marked decrease in life expectancy. His evidence was taken from studies of survival in hospitalized demented patients. Combining this evidence with available information on the prevalence of Alzheimer's disease, he concluded that this disorder may be the fourth or fifth most common cause of death in the United States. Although in Katzman's argument, Alzheimer's disease is a 'major killer', he pointed out that it was excluded as such from official statistics on causes of death, being supplanted by other acute events often occurring at the deaths of demented individuals. The situation Katzman described in the United States could reasonably be generalized to other developed countries. However, Katzman's argument has a possible weakness in that it was based on studies of survival in hospitalized cases. Such cases may be in worse general health than those which remain in the community.

To get an accurate view of the effects of dementing diseases on survival, we need follow-ups of cases identified in studies of the general population. Since the time of Katzman's editorial, a number of relevant studies have been published. Studies of survival with general population samples may deal with either incident or prevalent cases. Studies of incident cases are the most relevant because they assess the reduction in survival in individuals from when they are first developing a dementing disease. By contrast, prevalent cases may vary between mild and very advanced cases and will inevitably have a shorter survival than new cases. However, both types of studies support Katzman's conclusion that dementing diseases are killers. Schoenberg *et al.* (1981) assessed incident cases using a medical case register in the United States. Cases were therefore new only as far as medical attention was concerned. Table 6.1 shows the observed and expected survival in these cases. While dementing diseases did not reduce survival in the short term, they did so in the longer term, presumably because cases tend to die only after the disease is advanced. Treves *et al.* (1986), in Israel, also used a medical case register to study survival, but confined their attention to pre-senile cases of Alzheimer's disease. By 10 years after onset, survival was less than 15%, compared to an expectation of around 85%. The malignancy of the pre-senile disease is thus very high. The only other study of survival in incident cases is that of Nilsson (1984) in Sweden. He found reduced survival in cases appearing in a cohort followed from 70 to 79 years of age. However, the number of cases was small and the reduction consequently not statistically significant.

Table 6.1 Survival in dementia cases new to a medical case register in Rochester, Minnesota. Adapted from Schoenberg *et al.* (1981)

Time from registration (years)	Survival of cases (%)	Expected survival (%)
1	93	92
5	49	64
10	16	37

Studies showing reduced survival in prevalent cases are more numerous. Such studies have been reported from Britain (Bergmann, 1977; Maule *et al.*, 1984), Sweden (Åkesson, 1969; Rorsman *et al.*, 1985a), Denmark (Nielsen *et al.*, 1981), Iceland (Magnusson and Helgason, 1981) and Finland (Mölsä *et al.*, 1984). These studies have used various approaches for ascertaining prevalent cases and different methods of indexing survival. Therefore, it is impossible to make simple summary statements about survival in prevalent cases. However, as would be expected, survival is longer in mild cases than in moderate or severe ones (Nielsen *et al.* 1981; Maule *et al.*, 1984; Rorsman *et al.*, 1985a).

Although there is now compelling evidence for reduced survival in dementia, the existing studies are limited in that most deal with the dementia syndrome rather than specific dementing diseases. To find out about relative survival in specific dementing diseases, we are forced to supplement the small amount of data from general population studies with the results of hospital- and clinic-based studies.

6.2 RELATIVE SURVIVAL IN ALZHEIMER AND VASCULAR DEMENTIAS

Only two general population studies have examined relative surivival in Alzheimer and vascular dementias. Both of these used prevalent cases. The first study, by Åkesson (1969) in Sweden, found that vascular cases had poorer survival than Alzheimer cases. However, the numbers of each type of dementing disease were so small that not too much credence can be placed in the results. The other study was by Mölsä *et al.* (1984) in Finland. They had quite large numbers of cases and were able subsequently to carry out a neuropathological diagnosis for many of them (Mölsä *et al.*, 1988). Consistent with Åkesson (1969), this study also found that survival was worse for vascular dementias.

There have also been many hospital- and clinic-based studies comparing survival in Alzheimer and vascular dementias. These studies have generally measured survival from diagnosis or admission. Table 6.2 summarizes the results. Because of the varying methods of measuring

Table 6.2   Relative survival in Alzheimer and vascular dementias, as found in hospital- and clinic-based studies

Author(s)	Year	Source of cases	Point survival measured from	Dementing disease with worse survival
Roth	1955	Hospital	Admission	Alzheimer
Kidd	1962	Hospital	Admission	Alzheimer
Kay	1962	Hospital	Admission	Alzheimer for males, vascular for females
Shah *et al.*	1969	Hospital	Admission	Alzheimer
Varsamis *et al.*	1972	Hospital	Admission	No difference
Go *et al.*	1978	Hospital	Onset	Vascular
Duckworth *et al.*	1979	Hospital	Admission	Vascular
Blessed and Wilson	1982	Hospital	Admission	No difference
Christie	1982	Hospital	Admission	Vascular
Reding *et al.*	1984	Clinic	Diagnosis	Vascular
Barclay *et al.*	1985b	Clinic	Diagnosis	Vascular
Martin *et al.*	1987a	Clinic	Diagnosis	Vascular

survival, it is impossible to quantify the results of these studies beyond saying which dementing disease had worse survival. The findings are mixed, with some studies showing worse survival in Alzheimer cases and others in vascular cases. However, when studies are arranged chronologically, as in Table 6.2, an interesting pattern emerges, with the earlier studies showing a worse outcome for Alzheimer's disease and the later ones a worse outcome for vascular dementia. It is also notable that the early studies were based on hospital admission, whereas the most recent involve clinic cases. It is therefore likely that the recent studies saw cases at an earlier stage of their dementia.

A possible explanation for this pattern of results is that survival was worse for Alzheimer's disease in the 1950s and 1960s, but had improved relative to vascular cases by the 1980s. Alternatively, Alzheimer cases may reach services relatively later, or vascular cases relatively earlier, than was formerly the case. The possibility of historical changes of this sort is considered next.

6.3 HISTORICAL CHANGES IN SURVIVAL

Any historical change in survival of dementia cases is of great interest because it would lead to a corresponding change in prevalence. Gruenberg (1977) has argued that survival in many chronic diseases has increased this century because the terminal infections, such as pneumonia, which were often the immediate cause of death are now treatable. Indeed, mortality from pneumonia has continued to decline up to recent times, even for the very elderly (Manton, 1986). Although the development of effective treatments for infectious diseases like pneumonia was a great success, it has the adverse consequence of longer survival for the victims of chronic diseases. Gruenberg referred to these effects on chronic diseases as 'the failures of success'. Included amongst these 'failures' by Gruenberg was a longer survival of dementia cases. Gruenberg's evidence for longer survival came from an analysis of the Lundby study which was carried out from 1947 to 1972 in a rural area of southern Sweden. He compared the ten-year survival of cases identified in 1947 with cases identified in 1957. The 1957 cases had a survival similar to that of the general population, in contrast to the reduced survival of the 1947 cases. This was only a preliminary analysis of the Lundby data. Subsequently, Rorsman *et al.* (1985a) investigated mortality in the Lundby cohort over the full 25 years, from 1947 to 1972. When the first ten-year period was compared to the second 15-year period, the death rate in dementia cases was found to be lower in the second period, but by a statistically insignificant amount. Similarly, there was no significant change in the over-mortality of the dementia cases compared to mentally healthy controls. Later, Rorsman *et al.* (1985b) examined survival in

Alzheimer and vascular cases separately and found no significant change in survival for either group.

The Lundby study is unique in that it is the only general population survey to have continued long enough to detect historical changes. The only other evidence available on the issue comes from hospitalized cases. The hospital-based studies fall into two groups. The first consists of studies which have attempted to update early work in Britain by Roth (1955). Duckworth *et al.* (1979), Christie (1982) and Blessed and Wilson (1982), have all examined survival in recent hospital admissions using the same diagnostic criteria as Roth and compared their data with his earlier results. All studies found improved survival from time of admission and this improvement was greater for Alzheimer than vascular cases. However, all of these studies were carried out in different hospitals from Roth's. The study by Duckworth *et al.* (1979) was even carried out in a different country (Canada). Therefore historical changes have been confounded with hospital admission practices. The second group of hospital-based studies have looked at survival in the one hospital. This type of analysis has been carried out by Christie and Train (1984) in Britain for the periods 1957–1959 and 1974–1976, by Thompson and Eastwood (1981) in Canada for the period 1969–1978, and by Saugstad and Ødegård (1979) in Norway for the period 1950–1974. The results of these studies are, unfortunately, not consistent with the first group. Christie and Train (1984) did find longer survival in 1974–1976 than in 1957–1959, but this was only statistically significant for the very elderly (aged 85+). Furthermore, there was no differential improvement in survival between the Alzheimer and vascular patients. Thompson and Eastwood (1981) studied only Alzheimer patients and likewise showed no change in survival. However, their period of study (1969 – 1978) did not stretch as far back as Roth's early work on survival. To complicate the matter further, Saugstad and Ødegård (1979) found poorer survival over time for Alzheimer and vascular dementias in their Norwegian hospital. These conflicting results may, of course, be due to differing admission policies between hospitals. Given the lack of historical change in the Lundby study and the inconsistencies of the hospital-based studies, we can only conclude that there is presently no convincing evidence that survival of dementia cases has improved in recent decades.

6.4 AGE OF ONSET AND SURVIVAL

It has often been claimed that earlier-onset cases of Alzheimer's disease tend to have a faster progression than later-onset cases (e.g. Bondareff, 1983). This difference in progression of clinical changes should also be observed as a difference in survival. Earlier-onset cases are comparatively rare in the general population, so studies of the issue have been based on hospital and clinic series.

When looking at age effects, there are two contrasting influences. The more rampant course of earlier-onset cases might be expected to reduce survival. However, the younger age of these cases would tend to increase their survival. Indeed, better survival of younger cases has generally been found, whether survival is measured from onset (Larsson *et al.*, 1963; Go *et al.*, 1978; Heston, 1981; Seltzer and Sherwin, 1983; Diesfeldt *et al.*, 1986; Treves *et al.*, 1986) or from diagnosis (Heyman *et al.*, 1987). However, a couple of studies did not find such a difference. Barclay *et al.* (1985a) and Sayetta (1986) found no effect of age on survival. As might be expected, a rather different result emerges when the observed survival is corrected for expected survival, e.g. by expressing survival as a percentage of that expected. Then, the earlier-onset cases are generally found to fare more poorly (Larsson *et al.*, 1963; Go *et al.*, 1978; Seltzer and Sherwin, 1983; Barclay *et al.* 1985a; Diesfeldt *et al.*, 1986). The only exception to the general trend is the study by Treves *et al.* (1986), but this dealt with age-of-onset effects only amongst early-onset cases (aged 60 or less). In summary then, earlier-onset cases of Alzheimer's disease tend to have longer survival, but the disease has a more adverse effect on their life expectancy.

Nothing is known about the influence of age-of-onset in cases of vascular dementia.

6.5 SEX DIFFERENCES IN SURVIVAL

Because males have a shorter life expectancy than females, it might be expected that this difference also applies to cases with dementing diseases. In the only general population study of the issue, Rorsman *et al.* (1985a) found this to be so of cases for the dementia syndrome. Clinic- and hospital-based studies have also generally found worse survival in male cases of Alzheimer's disease (Kay, 1962; Larsson *et al.*, 1963; Heston, 1981; Barclay *et al.*, 1985; Diesfeldt *et al.*, 1986; Heyman *et al.*, 1987) and vascular dementia (Go *et al.*, 1978). The only exception was the study of Go *et al.* (1978) which found little sex difference in survival for Alzheimer cases.

The more theoretically interesting issue is whether the sexes differ in survival corrected for expectation. When this was done in the general population study by Rorsman *et al.* (1985a), demented men were still found to fare worse over the years 1947–1957, but there was little sex difference over the period 1957–1972. In the clinic- and hospital-based studies, male survival corrected for expectation was still worse for Alzheimer cases (Kay, 1962; Larsson *et al.*, 1963; Go *et al.*, 1978; Barclay *et al.*, 1985; Diesfeldt *et al.*, 1986), but the results are more mixed for vascular ones (Kay, 1962; Go *et al.*, 1978). This sex difference in survival helps explain why prevalence studies generally show a preponderance of females with Alzheimer's disease, but incidence studies show more mixed results (see Chapter 5). A higher female prevalence of Alzheimer's disease would result if there was no sex difference in incidence, but relatively better female survival.

6.6 ETHNIC AND REGIONAL DIFFERENCES

Ethnic differences in survival have been examined by Treves *et al.* (1986) in their study of the incidence of pre-senile Alzheimer's disease in Israel. These investigators found that incidence was higher in Jews of European and American origin compared to Jews of African and Asian origin. However, there was no difference in survival between the two groups, showing that the European and American cases were not more malignant.

Regional differences in survival were looked at in the US/UK Cross-National Project. This study found a higher prevalence and incidence of dementia in New York than London (Gurland *et al.*, 1983). A one-year follow-up of prevalent cases showed that those in New York had a higher mortality rate (33%) than those in London (0%). Since cases were identified using the same methodology in both cities, it is unlikely that the effect reflects case-finding differences. At present, this regional difference remains unexplained.

The final study on this topic compared survival of nursing home residents in New York and Tokyo (Vitaliano *et al.*, 1981). In both cities, survival from admission was found to be adversely affected by dementia. However, there was no difference in survival between dementing residents in the two cities. This was despite a presumed difference in the composition of the demented patients, with vascular dementia predominating in the Japanese cases. Whether this similarity in survival can be generalized to non-institutionalized cases is unknown. Certainly, differences in admission policies between countries could easily reduce or accentuate survival differences in the general population.

6.7 CAUSES OF DEATH IN DEMENTIA CASES

While Alzheimer's disease and vascular dementia are clearly malignant, as Katzman (1976) argued, they are often not recorded as the cause of death in affected individuals. Acute disorders immediately preceding death tend to supplant them. Several studies of dementia-related deaths in the general population have examined the immediate causes of death in such cases. Schoenberg *et al.* (1981) identified cases using a comprehensive medical case register in the United States. They found that most deaths in Alzheimer cases were due to respiratory disease, with cardiovascular disease the next most common factor. In vascular dementia cases, cardiovascular disease predominated as the immediate cause of death. Mölsä *et al.* (1984) in Finland followed up dementia cases identified in a prevalence study and found that bronchopneumonia was the immediate cause of death in over 70% of cases, with myocardial infarction and pulmonary embolism each accounting for a further 10%. Unfortunately, these researchers did not provide a breakdown of immediate cause of death by type of dementing disease. Consistent with the results from studies of the general population, bronchopneumonia has emerged as the major immediate cause of death in hospital- and clinic-based series of cases (Goodman, 1953; Varsamis *et al.*, 1972: Peck *et al.*, 1978; Saugstad and Ødegård, 1979; Sulkava *et al.*, 1983).

As discussed previously, Gruenberg (1977) has argued that the successful treatment of infectious diseases like pneumonia has had the effect of increasing the survival of dementia cases. While no clear evidence of a survival increase has been found, pneumonia might still have become less prominent as an immediate cause of death. The only data on this issue come from Saugstad and Ødegård's study of deaths in a Norwegian psychiatric hospital. They found that respiratory disease (mainly bronchopneumonia) was about 40 times as common a cause of death in dementia cases as in the general population. However, between 1950 and 1975, mortality from this cause declined only insignificantly. This finding provides indirect support for the conclusion that survival of dementia cases has not improved much over recent decades.

6.8 USE OF DEATH CERTIFICATES TO STUDY DEMENTIA MORTALITY

Carrying out epidemiological field studies of dementing diseases is expensive and difficult. Some researchers have attempted a short-cut by using death certificate data. Causes of death are routinely coded from death certificates in many countries and provide a ready source of data for epidemiological research. In most countries, only the underlying cause of death is officially recorded, but in some countries contributory causes are recorded as well. Dementia mortality will, of course, be much higher when contributory causes are included.

Mortality data have been used by several researchers to study dementing diseases. Chandra *et al.* (1986a), Aubert *et al.* (1987) and Newman and Bland (1987) have used death certificate data to study age and sex differences in mortality from dementing diseases. Chandra *et al.* (1986b) have also carried out a case-control study of co-morbidity in cases having a dementing disease listed on the death certificate, compared to controls which have other causes listed. However, probably the major and most controversial use of death certificate data has been to study regional differences in dementia mortality.

Mortality from dementia, as assessed through death certificates, shows major regional variation within countries. Some researchers believe that these are true differences and have proposed that local environmental factors are responsible. For example, Edwardson *et al.* (1986) in Britain have reported that the county of Northumberland has over twice the dementia mortality rate of the neighbouring county of Durham. They speculated that differences in the natural mineral content of soil and water and the use of aluminium to treat drinking water could be responsible. Because aluminium has no known biological function, but is found in the amyloid core of senile plaques and in tangle-bearing neurons, considerable interest has centred on the possible aetiological role of this element. Edwardson *et al.* (1986) pointed out that the dementia mortality difference between Northumberland and Durham is associated with a corresponding difference in the aluminium content of their water supplies. Norwegian researchers have also related regional differences in dementia mortality to the aluminium content of drinking water. Usually, aluminium is present at only low levels in drinking water, but its availability increases if the water is acidic. In much of Norway, acid rain has led to leaching of aluminium from the soil and into the water supply. Vogt (1986) divided southern Norway into five zones according to the aluminium concentration in their lakes and found that dementia mortality (as assessed through death certificates) increased across zones in line with the aluminium concentration. Flaten (1987) used a similar approach. He divided Norway into 193 geographical units and correlated the aluminium content of drinking water with dementia mortality. The correlation was low (0.23 for males and 0.27 for females), but statistically significant.

Although death certificates provide a convenient source of epidemiological data, there is evidence which questions their validity as far as dementing diseases are concerned. This evidence indicates that certified dementia mortality is a poor indicator of actual dementia mortality and is greatly influenced by death certification practices. If dementia mortality rates derived from death certificates were valid we might expect them to be relatively stable over time, particularly since there is no convincing evidence that incidence, survival or prevalence have changed markedly in recent decades. However, marked changes have been observed over quite short periods (i.e. a decade or less). Considerable increases in mortality from dementing diseases have been reported in Canada (Newman and Bland, 1987), the United States (Aubert *et al.*, 1987), Britain (Martyn and Pippard, 1988) and Australia (Jorm *et al.*, 1989). In Norway, where both underlying and contributory causes of death are recorded, there has been an increase in dementia as an underlying cause, but a decrease as a contributory cause (Flaten, 1989). Contrary to the trend for dementia, deaths from the vague cause of 'senility' have declined (Flaten, 1989; Jorm *et al.*, 1989; Martyn and Pippard, 1988). These changes are likely to be due to diagnostic fashion. One can only wonder about the influence of Katzman's (1976) editorial pointing out that Alzheimer's disease was long neglected as a cause of death and the generally greater knowledge of dementing disorders amongst medical practitioners.

There is other more direct evidence questioning the validity of death certificate data. Martyn and Pippard (1988) examined the death certificates of 117 patients who had been diagnosed as demented during life and found that pre-senile or senile dementia was recorded as the underlying cause of death in only 22% of cases and was mentioned at all on the death certificate in only 57%. Furthermore, they found that cases dying in psychiatric hospitals were more likely to have dementia on the death certificate than cases dying elsewhere. This finding suggested a possible explanation for regional variation in dementia mortality. When the map of dementia mortality in England and Wales was compared with one showing the location of large psychiatric hospitals, a remarkable degree of correspondence was apparent. Jorm *et al.* (1989), in Australia, have also found limitations in death certificate data. They found that mortality from dementia was similar in all the Australian states, except for Tasmania, which had a markedly higher rate. When people who were born in Tasmania but died elsewhere were compared with people who were born elsewhere but died in Tasmania, place of death was found to be a more important determinant of dementia mortality than place of birth. This difference implicated death certification practices in Tasmania. Jorm *et al.* then examined mortality within regions of Tasmania and found a very high rate in the north of the state. However, nearly half the death certifiiates in this region listing dementia as the underlying cause were found to be written by one medical practitioner working at a particular institution. Thus, the death certification practices of a single practitioner may have a considerable distorting influence on a whole region.

Although death certificates have provided useful data for the epidemiological study of many diseases, they are presently of limited use for dementing diseases. These diseases are often not recognized by medical practitioners while the patient is still alive (Williamson *et al.*, 1964; Parsons, 1965; Weyerer, 1983; O'Connor *et al.*, 1988) and, where they are recognized, may not be regarded as a cause of death. With greater knowledge of the diseases and their malignancy, death certificate data might eventually attain a degree of validity which makes them suitable for research purposes. The rapid rise in reported dementia mortality in several countries suggests that such a trend is occurring.

7 Psycho-social correlates

The hypotheses which lay people put forward to explain dementia are very often psycho-social in character. The deterioration of a relative may be attributed to an inactive lifestyle, too much stress, or certain pre-morbid intellectual and personality characteristics. Yet despite the public interest in psycho-social factors, they have received less attention from epidemiologists than genetic factors or toxic exposures. This chapter reviews what evidence there is on the role of socio-economic status, pre-morbid ability, life stress and personality in the genesis of dementia.

7.1 SOCIO-ECONOMIC STATUS

Socio-economic status (SES) is a construct which can be measured via occupation, income, education or some amalgam of these. All three indicators of SES are correlated, as would be expected, since education is a major determinant of occupation, which in turn determines income. Education is the most-used indicator of SES in studies of dementia. It is more easily placed on an ordinal scale than occupation and is less problematic for the elderly than income, which will be affected by retirement. Here, studies using any of these indicators will be reviewed as though they are equivalent.

Studies of SES have involved various levels of diagnostic specificity, ranging from measurement of cognitive impairment to diagnosis of specific dementing diseases. Most numerous have been studies of cognitive impairment. Kramer *et al.* (1985) and Weissman *et al.* (1985) in the USA have used the Mini-Mental State Examination (MMSE) to define cognitive impairment and found a marked educational gradient. In the Kramer *et al.* study, severe cognitive impairment was found in 12.5% of the least-educated group compared to only 1.6% of the most-educated. For Weissman *et al.* (1985) the corresponding range was from 6.1% to 0.2%. In China, Yu *et al.* (1989) found severe cognitive impairment in 11.4% of illiterates compared to only 0.4% of those with a college education. O'Connor *et al.* (1989b) in Britain have shown that cognitive impairment on the MMSE is related to both education and social class. In their elderly sample, cognitive impairment was found in 12% of those who left school after 15 compared to 23% of those who left before this age. For the higher social classes, cognitive impairment was present in 12%, compared to 24% for the lower social classes. Other studies have not used a cut-off to define cognitive impairment, but have simply correlated MMSE scores with education. Significant negative correlations have been reported by Holzer *et al.* (1984) and Fillenbaum *et al.* (1988) in the United States, by Escobar *et al.* (1986) with Spanish-speaking Americans, by Jorm *et al.* (1988a) in Australia, and by Li *et al.* (1989) in China.

Other screening instruments similarly correlate with indicators of SES. Using a continuous dementia scale, Gurland *et al.* (1983) found negative correlations with education and occupational status in both New York and London. Studies in the USA using a variety of screening tests have likewise found negative relationships with education (Kahn *et al.*, 1961; Pfeiffer, 1975; Scherr *et al.*, 1988) and occupational status (Scherr *et al.*, 1988). The existing evidence therefore uniformly supports the conclusion that low SES is associated with cognitive impairment.

The relationship with diagnosed dementia is less clear-cut, however. Kay *et al.* (1964b), in a study of community dwellers in England, found social class to be unassociated with the prevalence of organic mental disorders. By contrast, Lin *et al.* (1969) in Taiwan did find some association with social class and education, but his overall prevalence rates were so low that one must suspect less thorough case-finding than in other studies. Similarly, Dilling and Weyerer (1984) in Germany found a trend for dementia prevalence to be inversely related to social class, but the statistical reliability of the result is doubtful. The strongest relationship between education and diagnosed dementia has emerged in a study by Li *et al.* (1989) in China. This study is particularly interesting because a third of the elderly population was illiterate. Dementia was diagnosed in 2.2% of the illiterates, 1.4% of the semi-literates and 0.6% of those with primary or more education. However, age and sex are significantly correlated with illiteracy in China, it being more common in the very old and in women. When these two variables were statistically controlled, there was no significant relationship between dementia prevalence and education. The limited results available seem to support Gurland's (1981) conclusion that diagnosed dementia is more weakly associated with SES than is cognitive impairment. This presumably occurs because cognitive impairment includes life-long poor intellectual functioning as well as more recent cognitive decline. Life-long poor intellectual functioning is well known to be associated with low SES.

Only one study has examined the association between SES and specific dementing diseases. Sulkava (pers. commun.) in Finland has looked at the prevalence of dementing diseases in relation to education and income. He found that the prevalence of Alzheimer's disease was significantly lower in individuals with more than an elementary education. By contrast, there was no significant difference in the prevalence of vascular dementia between educational groups. When prevalence was examined by income, a similar relationship emerged. The prevalence of Alzheimer's disease was significantly lower in the higher income groups, but there was no corresponding difference with vascular dementia. Such results are difficult to explain.

There are, as well, several case-control studies of clinically-diagnosed Alzheimer's disease which have looked at SES differences. However, the interpretation of these is not as simple as with population surveys, because SES factors may influence selection into the study rather than the operation of a true risk factor. Cases coming to clinical attention may be socio-economically different from cases in the total population and controls who are willing to participate in a research study may likewise be different.

If SES is associated with prevalence of cognitive impairment or diagnosed dementia, the association could be with either incidence or survival. Unfortunately, no studies of SES correlates of incidence or survival have been done. However, there is some evidence concerning the relationship of SES to the course of Alzheimer's disease. Filley *et al.* (1985) followed cases of Alzheimer's disease over one year and quantified their rate of decline. Better-educated cases were found to deteriorate at the same rate as the more poorly-educated. Similarly, Berg *et al.* (1984) followed mild Alzheimer cases over one year and found that neither education nor social position differentiated those who remained mild from those who deteriorated further.

7.1.1 The problem of assessment bias

It is possible that associations with SES arise because of assessment or diagnostic procedures which are socio-culturally biased. The problem of assessment bias is a vexed one. To some, the observation of a difference between SES groups is, *ipso facto*, evidence of bias. This position has been most clearly stated by Kittner *et al.* (1986). They pointed out that diagnosis of dementia is often a two-stage process: a screening phase to detect poor cognitive functioning, and a diagnostic phase to identify the reasons for this poor functioning. If the screening phase is biased, then so will be the whole diagnostic process. Because screening tests have been shown to correlate with education, Kittner *et al.* argued that low scores will imply greater deterioration in a highly-educated person than in a less-educated person. To overcome this problem, they advocated that cognitive screening tests should be made more difficult for the well-educated person. This could be achieved by using different pass/tail cutting points for different levels of education. Kittner *et al.* went so far as to suggest that, in some cases, completely different screening tests might be appropriate for individuals with different SES backgrounds. A similar conclusion was reached by Escobar *et al.* (1986) who studied a Spanish-speaking American sample with the MMSE. After finding that educational level and ethnicity influenced scores, they concluded that 'the MMSE should be revised with items selected or re-weighted to diminish social and educational artifacts' (p. 613).

An opposing view has been argued by Berkman (1986). She pointed out that SES indicators are associated with many diseases and, in some cases, this has provided important clues to aetiology. If there were a genuine association between educational attainment and dementia incidence, then adjusting screening tests to remove the correlation with education would hinder research on an important risk factor. Since it is unknown whether the correlation with education is a reflection of test bias or a genuine risk factor, Berkman argued that it is premature to adjust screening test scores to remove the association. However, she did admit that some part of the association with education is probably due to pre-morbid characteristics rather than to brain pathology.

The issue of test bias is a familiar one to developers of psychological and educational tests. Whenever any group difference is found on a test, the issue arises of whether it is a true difference or due to bias. Techniques have been developed to detect bias in tests or in particular items within tests. These techniques have been well summarized by Jensen (1980) and Reynolds (1982). Psychometricians regard a test as biased if there are differences in the validity of the test which are

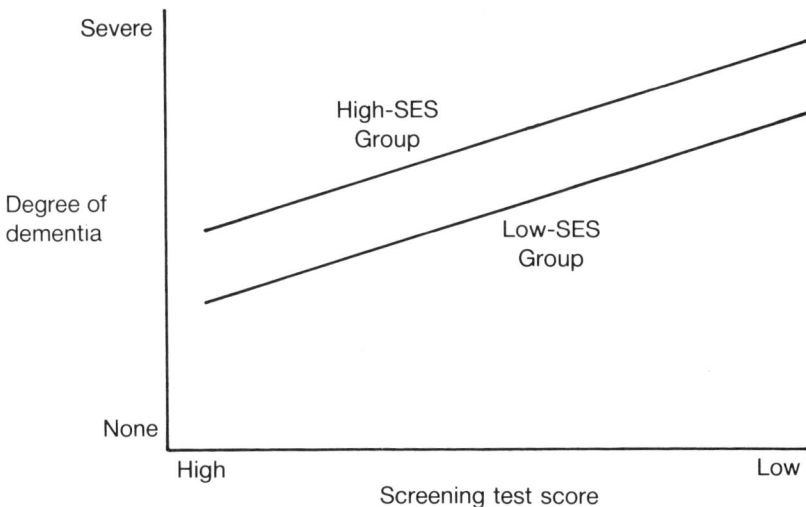

Figure 7.1 Hypothetical regression lines predicting degree of dementia from screening test scores using a socio-economically biased test.

associated with group membership. In the case considered here, group membership is defined by educational attainment, occupational status or income.

There are several ways of assessing the validity of a test. As far as detecting bias is concerned, the best method of establishing validity is to predict some criterion or 'gold standard'. For each SES group, a regression line is calculated for predicting the criterion from test scores. If the test is unbiased, the regression lines for the high and low SES groups should not differ in any way. If a difference between groups is found in the slope, intercept or standard error of estimate of the respective regression lines, then the test is biased. Figure 7.1 shows the example of regression lines which differ in intercept. This situation would result if a given screening test score corresponded to greater dementia in a high-SES person than in a low-SES person. In suggesting that screening tests should be corrected for education, Kittner *et al.* (1986) were implying such a situation.

In practice, little evidence has been collected on group differences in predictive validity of screening tests. Part of the problem is that there is no gold standard to use as a criterion. Clinical diagnosis and daily living skills have been used as criteria for establishing predictive validity, but this assumes that such criterion measures are themselves unbiased. Despite the lack of a gold standard, a few studies have attempted to assess bias in screening instruments by examining predictive validity in different groups. In an important study of the issue, Anthony *et al.* (1982) used clinical diagnosis as the criterion to evaluate educational bias in the MMSE. While the test performed well overall, there were many false positives for elderly people with less than nine years of education. Thus, the test appeared to be a biased predictor of dementia for the poorly educated. Anthony *et al.* examined various modifications of the MMSE, such as altering cut-offs and eliminating certain items, but were unable to improve the overall performance of the test. They concluded that new items which are less sensitive to education might need to be devised.

Other studies, using activities of daily living as the criterion, have found no evidence of bias in screening instruments. Gurland (1981) examined bias in the Mental Status Questionnaire as part of the US/UK Cross-National Project. He found that dependency rose as a function of Mental Status scores to about the same degree in high- and low-educated groups. Thus, 77% of people scoring 4+ on the Mental Status Questionnaire were dependent in both the high- and low-education groups, yet scores this poor were found in 17% of the low-education group compared to only 5% of the high-education group. Jorm *et al.* (1988a) also used daily living skills as a criterion to evaluate the predictive validity of the MMSE in an Australian community sample.

The more-educated group performed better on both the MMSE and the activities of daily living assessment and the regression line predicting daily living skills from MMSE scores did not differ as a function of education. These results are counter-evidence for education bias and are inconsistent with the conclusions of Anthony *et al.* (1982). An obvious explanation for the discrepancy is in terms of the different type of criterion measures used – clinical diagnoses vs. daily living skills. It could be argued that Anthony *et al.*'s (1982) clinical diagnosis was biased in favour of the less educated, or that the assessments of daily living skills used by Gurland (1981) and Jorm *et al.* (1988a) were as equally biased as cognitive screening tests. Without a gold standard, there is no resolution to this issue. All we can say is that a screening instrument is or is not biased when judged against a particular arbitrary criterion. If the purpose of a screening instrument is to predict who needs practical assistance in daily living because of cognitive impairment, then screening tests may be unbiased. If, however, the purpose is to select individuals who have a high probability of being diagnosed as demented by a clinician, then these tests may at the same time be biased. To complicate matters even further, an assessment may also differ in the extent of bias depending on the particular diagnostic criteria against which it is judged. For example, DSM-III-R criteria for dementia require the presence of various kinds of cognitive **impairment** whereas ICD-10 research diagnostic criteria specifically require cognitive **decline**. Since screening tests typically assess cognitive impairment rather than cognitive decline, they could conceivably be biased with ICD-10 dementia as the criterion, but not with DSM-III-R dementia.

While most research on bias has concentrated on screening tests, there may also be bias in clinical diagnosis. The problem of finding a criterion for establishing predictive validity is even more difficult for clinical diagnoses than for screening tests. Because unselected series of neuropathologically diagnosed elderly are not feasible, future course of the disorder remains the only available criterion. Bergmann *et al.* (1971) used this approach in a study of cases of 'suspected chronic brain syndrome' identified in a community survey. They found that some of these suspected cases had improved to such a degree at follow-up that the original diagnosis of organic impairment was unlikely. These im-proved subjects were more likely to come from the lowest social classes than those who progressed. On a dementia screening test, the subjects who were normal at follow-up were found actually to have poorer initial scores than those who deteriorated. It appears that these individuals had life-long poor cognitive functioning. Thus, both the clinical diagnosis and the screening test gave biased results for low social class individuals. Diagnosis of moderate and severe cases did not, however, appear to be biased in the same way, because there was no association between dementia prevalence and social class (Kay *et al.*, 1964b). The potential for diagnostic bias may therefore be greater with mild dementia.

Although predictive validity methods are, in principle, the ideal for detecting bias, other internal validity methods have been proposed (Jensen, 1980; Reynolds, 1982). These involve splitting a sample into two groups, e.g. high- and low-SES, and separately assessing the internal psychometric characteristics of the screening test. For example, the order of item difficulties should be the same for the two groups, as should the structure of the test as shown by principal components or factor analysis. Jorm *et al.* (1988a) have applied such internal validity methods to the MMSE, but found no evidence of bias. Such methods deserve wider use in researching the issue of bias in screening tests.

7.1.2 Possible mechanisms of an SES association

Assuming that there is an association between SES and dementia incidence which is not due to assessment bias, how could such an association arise? It is unlikely that SES could be a direct cause of dementia. Rather, it must be a proxy for some other variable which is involved in aetiology. One possibility is that SES is related to lifestyle preferences and occupational exposures which play a role in the aetiology of dementing diseases. For example, low SES people tend to have higher blood pressure, poorer control of hypertension and higher serum cholesterol, and these factors may play a role in vascular dementia (Berkman, 1986). With Alzheimer's disease, less is known about SES-related risk factors, but similar associations are plausible.

The second possibility is that high-SES people have a greater resistance to the effects of dementing diseases. This could arise if high-SES people have greater cognitive or neural reserves and can lose more neurons before showing ill-effects in daily living. SES then becomes a proxy for pre-morbid intellectual attributes. A third possibility is that high-SES people seek more stimulating environments in which cognitive skills are continuously practised. When cognitive skills are not used, they may waste away and make a person more prone to the effects of organic brain change. The possible effects of pre-morbid ability and a stimulating environment merit special consideration and are therefore discussed separately.

7.2 PRE-MORBID ABILITY

There are several possible ways in which pre-morbid ability might influence dementia occurrence. The possibilities can be conveniently considered in terms of Roth's (1986) threshold model of dementia. According to this model, plaques and tangles exist in the brains of normal aged individuals as well as in Alzheimer's disease. The differen-

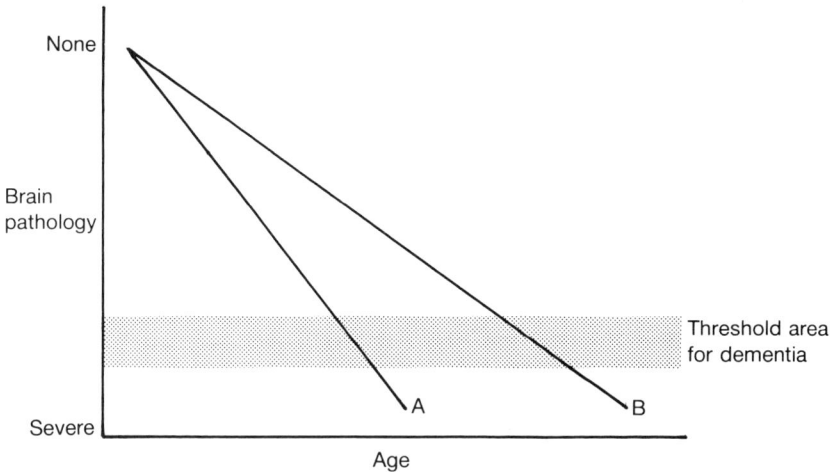

Figure 7.2   Threshold model of dementia showing ways in which pre-morbid ability might have an effect. Adapted from Mortimer (1988). For explanation of A and B, see text.

tiation between them is quantitative rather then qualitative. Dementia results when the extent of neuropathological changes exceeds a critical threshold. Mortimer (1988) has argued that pre-morbid ability has its influence on dementia by affecting the threshold for becoming a case. As shown in Figure 7.2, the threshold may be regarded as a fuzzy area rather than a fixed line. The same degree of brain pathology may have different implications for persons of high or low pre-morbid ability because of their different potential for compensation. Mortimer's view implies that pre-morbid ability does not affect the underlying neuro-pathology, but only the person's capacity to cope with the demands of daily life given a particular degree of pathology. Another implication is that the influence of pre-morbid ability will be seen with mild dementia but not with moderate or severe conditions.

In contrast to Mortimer's view, it could also be argued that pre-morbid ability has a direct influence on the rate of brain deterioration and cognitive decline. This possibility is represented in Figure 7.2 by the lines A and B. Persons of high pre-morbid ability might decline at a slower rate (line B) than persons of low pre-morbid ability (line A). The two views of how pre-morbid ability might have an effect are not, of course, mutually exclusive.

To evaluate adequately the role of pre-morbid ability requires longi-tudinal studies spanning decades. Regrettably, such studies are rare. The only study to address the issue is a 20-year longitudinal study of ageing twins (La Rue and Jarvik, 1987). Between 1946 and 1949, 268 twins with an average age of 70 were assessed on cognitive tests. From 1966 to 1968, 64 of these were examined psychiatrically when they were at an average age of 84. The cognitive tests were also repeated at this time. Twenty-eight of the 64 subjects were judged to have dementia of mild to severe degree. When the cognitive scores from 20 years earlier were examined, the now demented subjects were found to have done worse than the non-demented. Both groups declined over the 20-year interval, but the demented ones declined more. These relationships held even with the influence of education statistically removed. Because the interval of 20 years is much longer than the typical duration of dementias of old age, these results support the view that low pre-morbid ability is a risk factor for dementia. However, whether the influence of pre-morbid ability was via the threshold for caseness, or was due to differences in brain deterioration, is impossible to say.

Direct observation of brain ageing in people of high and low pre-morbid ability is presently not possible. However, there is some animal research to suggest that pre-morbid attributes can affect ageing of the brain. It is well known that a restricted environment during development can adversely affect brain function in experimental animals. However, Meaney *et al.* (1988) have recently shown that early environmental influences can attenuate deficits associated with ageing. They compared rats which had been handled in infancy with non-handled rats. The two groups of rats were studied during adulthood for hippocampal cell loss and spatial memory deficits. While the number of hippocampal neurones and spatial memory ability did not differ between handled and non-handled rats at six months of age, marked differences were found at 24 months. Thus, the early environmental manipulation seemed to affect aspects of the ageing process. It is plausible that similar effects could occur in human ageing. Pre-morbid ability might reflect early environmental advantages or disadvantages which also have an effect on the ageing brain.

There is also some neuropathological evidence on the human brain to support a protective role of pre-morbid neuronal reserve. Katzman *et al.* (1988) did a neuropathological study of a group of nursing home residents, most of whom died over the age of 80. They found a subgroup with the neuropathological features of mild Alzheimer's disease, but no cognitive impairment. When this subgroup was compared to demented subjects with Alzheimer's disease, they were found to have larger brains and a greater number of large neurones. Katzman *et al.* speculated that the subjects with preserved cognitive function may have had a greater neuronal reserve which gave them resistance to the effects of Alzheimer's disease. Another explanation is, however, possible. These subjects may simply have escaped the shrinkage and loss of large neurones which may accompany Alzheimer's disease.

7.2.1 Implications of an association with pre-morbid ability

If high pre-morbid ability does indeed have a protective effect in old age, this might produce a cohort effect in the incidence of dementia. This cohort effect could come about because of rising intelligence levels this century. Flynn (1984) has reviewed American studies which have established norms for intelligence tests and found evidence of consistent gains in scores over a period of 64 years. The total gain was 13.8 IQ points – almost one standard deviation. Later, Flynn (1987) confirmed this trend with data from 14 nations. The reason for the increase is unknown, but there is some evidence that it is due to rising levels of education (Teasdale and Owen, 1987). Although there is presently no convincing evidence of a change in dementia incidence over time (see Chapter 5), the evidence of rising intelligence comes from studies of children and young adults who have not yet reached old age. If rising intelligence were to reduce the incidence of dementia, the effect may not become apparent until the next century.

7.3 ENVIRONMENTAL STIMULATION IN LATER LIFE

An active and stimulating life is commonly believed to prevent cognitive decline in old age. There is, in fact, some good evidence that environmental restriction is related to cognitive impairment in the elderly. Huppert and Elliott (cited in Huppert, 1988) have reported a community survey of adults in Britain in which they were given an unexpected memory test for material earlier in the interveiw. Amongst elderly retired subjects, they found that educational qualifications and leisure activities had an interactive effect on memory performance. Number of leisure activities was related to memory performance for those with no educational qualifications, but there was no relationship for those with a qualification. This effect held even when IQ was controlled. In fact, those elderly adults who participated in several leisure activities performed as well as the more qualified, suggesting that a stimulating life may offset the disadvantage associated with poor education.

Of course, it is difficult to draw conclusions about a causal role of environmental stimulation from cross-sectional data. Failure to seek a stimulating environment could equally be a consequence of early cognitive decline as much as a cause. However, there is some animal research demonstrating the plausibility of a causal role. Cummins *et al.* (1973) reared rats in either a stimulating environment (containing toys) or a deprived one. The stimulated rats were found to have heavier brains and better maze-learning skill in adulthood. However, when the rats were old, they were given practice with mazes and this was found to increase the brain weights of the deprived rats, but not the stimulated ones. In fact, the maze-learning experience nearly abolished the brain-weight advantage of the rats who had had a stimulating environment in early life. The findings of Cummins *et al.* (1973) fit well with the suggestion by Huppert and Elliott (Huppert, 1988) that a stimulating life during retirement can offset the effects of earlier environmental disadvantage.

There is also some longitudinal human data supporting a causal role for environmental stimulation. Schaie (1984) followed a group of adults in the United States from middle to old age (from an average age of 46 years to 67 years). His findings showed that attitudinal flexibility, the maintenance of an engaged lifestyle and the absence of family dissolution are important in maintaining cognitive skills into old age. In a later study, Schaie and Willis (1986) selected groups of individuals who had shown declining cognitive skills over a 14-year period and attempted to re-train these skills. Using a five-hour training programme, they found that specific skills could be improved, but in less than half the subjects was there a return to previous levels. Older adults who had declined were found to benefit more from training than those who had remained stable, supporting the view that disuse of cognitive skills had contributed to the decline.

While these studies provide some evidence for a role of environmental stimulation in mild cognitive loss associated with ageing, they do not address its role in dementia. However, the longitudinal study by La Rue and Jarvik (1987) provided some supporting evidence for such a role. They followed a group of twins from 1947 to 1967 and classified them as demented or non-demented in 1967. When activity ratings for the two groups in 1947 were examined, the subsequently demented cases were found to be less active in physical, household and creative pursuits. However, when the influences of age and education were statistically controlled, these differences disappeared. The only statistically significant predictor of later dementia was passive activities. These included attendance at movies, sports, listening to the radio, reading, or watching television. The latter three activities tended to be the most common. Given the 20-year gap between the assessment of activities and the diagnosis of dementia, it is unlikely that this difference reflected early signs of dementia.

It seems implausible that lack of environmental stimulation could be a cause of the neuropathological changes seen in dementing disorders. It is more likely to have a contributory role by enhancing or retarding the cognitive effects of such changes.

7.4 LIFE STRESS

Stress has been claimed to be a risk factor for several chronic diseases and is frequently suggested by lay people as a cause of dementing diseases. Stress as a potential risk factor has also received some attention from dementia researchers.

Several studies have looked at the frequency of potentially stressful life events in the histories of Alzheimer cases versus controls. In three well-designed case-control studies the evidence on life events has been completely negative (French *et al.*, 1985; Amaducci *et al.*, 1986; Chandra *et al.*, 1987a). The only positive evidence comes from a study by Amster and Krauss (1974) which compared 25 cases of organic brain syndrome with 25 controls and found more stressful life events in cases during the five years preceding onset. However, the fact that studies with much larger sample sizes have not confirmed the result casts doubt on its reliability. Because risk factor information on cases is necessarily provided by informants, more stressful life events could easily be recalled in line with the informant's own preconceptions.

Another way of evaluating the effects of previous life stress is to look for its products (psychiatric disorders) rather than the frequency of presumed stressors (life events). Case-control studies by Heyman *et al.* (1984) and Soininen and Heinonen (1982) have found no excess of previous psychiatric disorders in Alzheimer cases. Similarly, a community survey by Kay *et al.* (1964b) and a psychiatric hospital study by Larsson *et al.* (1963) found that dementia cases do not have a higher lifetime prevalence of serious psychiatric disorders. By contrast, four case-control studies have found previous depression to be more common in Alzheimer cases than controls (Barclay *et al.*, 1985c; French *et al.*, 1985; Shalat *et al.*, 1987; Broe *et al.*, 1990). However, this difference seems to be attributable to an early manifestation of Alzheimer's disease (Broe *et al.*, 1990). It is known that depression can be a precursor of dementing disorders. For example, Reding *et al.* (1985) followed a group of elderly depressed patients, thought not to be demented, over a period of three years and found that around half of them went on to become clearly demented. Depression occurring in the years immediately preceding onset of a dementia disorder is better regarded as a prodromal feature rather than a risk factor.

Generally then, the evidence on life stress as a factor in Alzheimer's disease is negative. By contrast, there is no evidence presently available on its role with vascular dementia. However, because of the problem of 'effort after meaning' in the recall of informants, prospective studies of the issue are needed with both major dementing diseases.

7.5 PERSONALITY

Very little work has been done on pre-morbid personality as a risk factor. Two case-control studies of Alzheimer's disease have looked at the frequency of Type A personality in cases and controls (Amaducci *et al.*, 1986; Chandra *et al.*, 1987a). Type A individuals are characterized by time urgency and impatience, competitiveness and ambition, need for achievement, poor frustration tolerance, high occupational involvement and hostility. There is some evidence that such individuals are at higher risk for developing coronary heart disease. However, in the case-control studies of Alzheimer's disease, no association has emerged.

Other pre-morbid personality traits have not yet been investigated. Initial research in this area might do well to assess the role of the 'big two' personality traits; extraversion and neuroticism (trait anxiety). These have emerged most consistently in psychometric studies of personality questionnaires and can be reliably measured by informant reports as well as self report. These traits could conceivably be linked with different lifestyles which in turn are risk factors for dementing diseases. As with life stress, prospective studies will be necessary for any definitive answers because of effort after meaning in any retrospective reports by informants.

8 Risk factors for Alzheimer's disease

The study of risk factors for Alzheimer's disease was almost non-existent a decade ago, but is now a flourishing area of research, important because of its implications for the prevention of the disease. Public health campaigns for disease prevention usually take as their starting point the modification of risk factors. A great diversity of potential risk factors have been studied, many of them appearing in only one or two studies and failing to yield positive results. This chapter reviews only those factors which have been consistently researched or have some theoretical basis for their plausibility.

The predominant methodology used to discover risk factors for Alzheimer's disease is the case-control study. In such studies, clinically diagnosed cases are compared with controls for differences in past exposures. The strengths and weaknesses of the case-control study are fully discussed in Chapter 3. Case-control studies yield an odds ratio for exposure to a risk factor. This gives the odds of disease in individuals exposed to a potential risk factor divided by the odds of disease in non-exposed individuals. It can be used as an approximation to the relative risk, which is the incidence of disease in exposed individuals divided by the incidence in non-exposed. The relative risk tells how many more times an exposed individual is likely to develop the disease than a non-exposed individual. The odds ratio and relative risk can be used interchangeably as measures of the strength of association between a risk factor and the disease.

The evidence on risk factors for Alzheimer's disease is often mixed, with some studies showing significant associations which are not replicated in others. The traditional approach is to conclude that an association has been established only if it has been consistently replicated. However, weak associations will not produce consistently significant results unless researchers have used very large sample sizes. The approach adopted here is to concentrate more on the size of the association across studies rather than on the statistical significance of individual results. Associations which are consistently positive indicate that a true risk factor is operating, even if statistical significance is not achieved in most studies. The present approach therefore combines some of the features of meta-analysis (see Chapter 3) with the traditional literature review.

Risk factors for Alzheimer's disease can be conveniently grouped in terms of broad themes. Here, the research is summarized under the headings of socio-demographic characteristics, familial and genetic factors, birth factors and fertility, occupational and recreational exposures, previous illnesses and injuries, medical procedures, medication use, personal habits, and diet.

8.1 SOCIO-DEMOGRAPHIC CHARACTERISTICS

Included here are age, sex, country of residence and ethnicity. The effects of these variables on the incidence of Alzheimer's disease was discussed in Chapter 5. To summarize, old age is undoubtedly the strongest risk factor for Alzheimer's disease, although incidence may level-off in extreme old age. With sex, the incidence studies are inconsistent, with some showing a higher male incidence and others a higher female incidence. Few data are available on country of residence and ethnicity; however, a higher incidence of dementia has been reported in New York than London (Gurland *et al.*, 1983) and the incidence of early-onset Alzheimer's disease has been reported to be higher in Israeli Jews of European and American origin compared to those of African or Asian origin (Treves *et al.*, 1986).

8.2 GENETIC AND FAMILIAL FACTORS

There are a number of potential risk factors for Alzheimer's disease which are of a genetic nature. Three that have generated a reasonable amount of research are Down's syndrome, fingerprint patterns and handedness. It has also been suggested that Alzheimer's disease tends to be associated with a family history of certain diseases. The diseases which have been researched most thoroughly are Alzheimer's disease itself, Down's syndrome and haematological malignancies. A family history of such diseases might reflect the operation of genetic influences. However, a common environmental exposure is also a possibility.

8.2.1 Down's syndrome

Adults with Down's syndrome appear to have a greatly increased risk of dying with Alzheimer neuropathology. Struwe (1929) was the first to describe senile plaques in the brains of individuals with Down's syndrome, and there have been many similar reports of Alzheimer neuropathology since then. These reports have been reviewed by Oliver and Holland (1986). Most studies have involved small samples, the exceptions being studies by Malamud (1972) and Wisniewski *et al.* (1985). Malamud (1972) studied the brains of 131 Down's individuals, 35 of whom were aged over 40, and found that all individuals dying over this age had Alzheimer neuropathology. Wisniewski *et al.* (1985) studied 100 individuals and found that all of the 49 dying over 30 years of age had plaques and tangles. Both studies found Alzheimer neuropathology in some individuals as young as the second decade of life. On the basis of these studies, it is now generally accepted that nearly all individuals with Down's syndrome over the age of 35 or 40 have the neuropathological features of Alzheimer's disease. Down's syndrome has also been found to involve a cholinergic deficiency like that seen in Alzheimer's disease (Yates *et al.*, 1980), with a reduction in the enzymes choline acetyltransferase and acetylcholinesterase.

Since Alzheimer neuropathology is highly predictive of dementia in non-Down's individuals, it might be expected that dementia would invariably be present in Down's syndrome from middle-age onwards. However, dementia has been observed in only a minority of cases. For example, in Wisniewski *et al.*'s (1985) study only 15 of the 56 individuals with Alzheimer neuropathology had a history of dementia. While the demented individuals were found to have higher densities of plaques and tangles than the non-demented, the latter still had sufficient densities to qualify as Alzheimer's disease cases by standard criteria for neuropathological diagnosis. Because diagnosis of dementia was retrospective in Wisniewski *et al.*'s study, it is possible that some cases were missed. However, direct observations of cognitive and daily living skills in older Down's individuals also suggest that deterioration is far from the norm.

A number of studies have compared Down's individuals of various ages with non-Down's mentally retarded controls. If Down's syndrome involves dementia in middle and old age, then the Down's cases should show greater age-related deficits than the non-Down's controls. In an early study, Dalton *et al.* (1974) matched 20 Down's to 20 non-Down's mental retardates for age group. They found that the old Down's group (aged 44–58) had greater deficits on a visual retention test than either the young Down's or the control retardates. However, they found no greater deficits on visual matching, digit span or non-verbal intelligence. Later, Thase *et al.* (1984) compared 165 Down's to 163 age-matched mentally retarded controls. They found the Down's subjects to have greater age-related deficits on interviewer ratings of attention span, co-operation, lability and apathy. However, impairments were most evident in subjects aged over 50 years. The only objective cognitive test to show such an effect was digit span. Several other cognitive tests did not show significantly greater ageing decrements in Down's subjects. Silverstein *et al.* (1986) matched over 400 Down's subjects to non-Down's retarded controls and assessed them on 62 rating items covering motor, independent living, social, emotional, cognitive, communication and vocational domains. They found only three items for which the Down's subjects had greater cognitive decline with age: rolling and sitting, crawling and walking, and eating. Those items were worse only in the oldest age groups (60–69 years). In the largest study of this type, Zigman *et al.* (1987) matched 2144 Down's individuals to 4172 developmentally disabled controls. Assessments were carried out using behavioural scales which assessed activities of daily living and cognitive skills. Down's subjects showed more age-related deficits in both areas. With activities of daily living, Down's subjects only did worse than controls from age 60 onwards, while for cognitive skills they were worse from age 50 onwards. The deficit in the oldest Down's individuals was found to be due to a subgroup with very low scores rather than a small deficit in all individuals.

The above studies used cross-sectional age comparisons and so confounded ageing effects with cohort differences. It may be that older Down's represent a survival elite because the more handicapped died younger. Also, most studies are carried out on institutionalized populations and, because of changed practices in the care of the mentally retarded, more able Down's of the younger generation may be found living in the community rather than in institutions. Such effects may serve to reduce age differences in performance. The way to overcome such problems is to do longitudinal studies. Although no longitudinal studies of ageing in Down's syndrome have been carried out, a number of researchers have used psychological test data collected over many years to assess longitudinal changes. Fisher and Zeaman (1970) studied the growth and decline of intelligence in retardates using a 'semi-longitudinal' method. They took intelligence test data from subjects tested at least twice and connected each subject's points by straight lines. The slopes of these lines were then averaged within age intervals to get the typical course of intellectual change for that age period. These average slopes were made continuous by interconnecting them, so that a smooth curve resulted. When Down's and non-Down's retardates were compared, there was little difference in the shape of the curves. However, the curves were derived only up to age 48, so it is possible they could diverge after that age. In another retrospective study, Berry *et al.* (1984) reported on 42 Down's individuals tested an average of six years apart. These individuals were participants in a non-institutional rehabilitation programme. Significant improvements were found on cognitive tests and daily living skills, but the average ages at the two testings were only 21 and 27 years respectively. Some evidence of decline was found in a study by Hewitt *et al.* (1985). They studied intelligence test records of 23 institutionalized Down's individuals aged

50 or over. Between two and 11 previous assessments were available for each of these subjects. Decline was found in 15 cases, an increase in seven, and no change in one. Seven had lost more than one year in mental age, but staff reported behavioural deterioration in only three cases.

Taking all this evidence together, there is some indication of a greater age-related decline in Down's syndrome than in other mental retardates. However, the decline is far less serious, and occurs at a later age (from 50 onwards), than the neuropathology would indicate.

Several explanations are possible for this puzzling discrepancy. Firstly, as Oliver and Holland (1986) point out, the Alzheimer neuropathology may not be present in the elderly Down's individuals with no dementia. The view that all Down's over 35 or 40 have Alzheimer neuropathology is based on autopsies of those dying. If Alzheimer neuropathology was a contributing factor in the early deaths of these individuals, then they may not be representative of those who remain alive. Without an *in vivo* diagnostic test, it is impossible to know whether the neuropathology is present in living elderly individuals with Down's syndrome. Nevertheless, even those with confirmed neuropathology at autopsy often do not exhibit dementia before death.

A second possibility, also pointed out by Oliver and Holland (1986), is that the mental handicap of Down's syndrome is in fact partly due to dementia. It may be that the Alzheimer's disease begins affecting the brain before plaques and tangles are seen, so that the first effects occur during development. These effects come to be labelled as part of the mental handicaps of Down's syndrome, rather than part of the dementing process. However, if the dementia began this early then progressive deterioration would be expected from an early age when, in fact, continued mental development has been observed during the third decade of life in Down's syndrome (Fisher and Zeaman, 1970; Berry *et al.*, 1984).

A third possibility is that plaques and tangles vary in their effect depending on the neuronal substrate. The neuronal architecture of Down's individuals may differ in such a way that plaques and tangles do not interfere with function as readily. Since there is currently little understanding of how plaques and tangles do interfere with neuronal function, this possibility cannot be evaluated.

Finally, it is possible that plaques and tangles are not the central lesions in Alzheimer's disease. Although plaque and tangle counts are correlated with dementia severity in Alzheimer's disease, the relationship is by no means perfect. There may be some unknown lesion accounting for the dementia, with plaques and tangles being an epiphenomenon. In aged Down's individuals, the plaques and tangles may be present to a greater degree than the unknown lesion. Wisniewski and Rabe (1986) have shown that, amongst Down's individuals with Alzheimer neuro-pathology, the demented have a greater density of plaques and tangles than the non-demented. This observation has led them to suggest that the threshold for dementia is greater in Down's syndrome, with a greater density of plaques and tangles being required to produce clinically significant impairments. However, why there should be a higher threshold in Down's syndrome is unclear. If anything, the lower cognitive and neural reserves of Down's individuals should make them more susceptible to the effects of any brain lesions rather than less so.

8.2.2 Fingerprint patterns

It has long been known that individuals with Down's syndrome are more likely to have certain handprint and fingerprint patterns. The parents of Down's children also tend to have these patterns (Loesch, 1981). Weinreb (1985) examined fingerprints in Alzheimer's disease to see if there was a similar association. He compared 50 clinically-diagnosed cases, covering a wide range of ages, with 50 controls. In the cases, 82% of the fingerprint patterns were found to be ulnar loops compared to only 54% for the controls. Earlier studies of Down's syndrome had shown a 78% frequency of ulnar loops compared to 57% in control samples. In Weinreb's (1985) study, 72% of the Alzheimer cases were found to have eight or more ulnar loops on the ten fingers compared to 26% of controls, making this a highly discriminating feature. Later, Weinreb (1986) was able to replicate these findings on a new sample.

Studies by other researchers have, however, had more mixed results, with two achieving partial replication and two others completely failing to replicate Weinreb's findings. Seltzer and Sherwin (1986) found ulnar loops on 61% of the fingers of cases compared to 56% of controls. This is a small and statistically non-significant difference. However, when the cases were divided into early- and late-onset groups using a dividing age of 65 years, the early-onset group was found to have ulnar loops on 69% of fingers compared to 51% for late-onset cases. The frequency of ulnar loops in early-onset cases was significantly higher than for controls or late-onset cases. Individuals with eight or more ulnar loops were found to comprise 51% of the early-onset cases compared to only 17% of the late-onset ones. Although the early-onset cases had a higher frequency of ulnar loops, this was still lower than Weinreb's (1985) report of 72% with eight or more ulnar loops. Since Weinreb's cases were of both early and late onset, his strong results were not exactly replicated. Later, Ghidoni *et al.* (1987) found significantly more ulnar loops in Alzheimer patients, but this was only true of males; no difference was found for females. They also found an association between frequency of ulnar loops and family history of dementia in their control group. It is notable that Weinreb's (1985, 1986) studies were with predominantly male samples, while Seltzer and Sherwin's (1986) sample consisted entirely of males.

Other studies have entirely failed to replicate Weinreb's findings. Luxenberg *et al.* (1988) compared 56 clinically-diagnosed cases with 112 matched controls, but found no difference in frequency of ulnar loops or other patterns characteristic of Down's syndrome. Dividing the cases by age of onset or sex did not alter the negative findings. Podrabinek *et al.* (1988) compared 34 cases with 20 controls and similarly found no difference in frequency of ulnar loops. However, their sample was entirely female.

If it proves to be replicable, the raised frequency of ulnar loops in Alzheimer's disease provides another link with Down's syndrome. In studies of parents with Down's children it has been suggested that those with Down's-like patterns are undetected mosaics. That is, they carry some cells with trisomy of chromosome 21. If mosaics were also at increased risk for early-onset Alzheimer's disease, as suggested by Rowe *et al.* (1989), there would be a plausible mechanism for an association with ulnar loops.

8.2.3 Handedness

An association between handedness and Alzheimer's disease was first proposed by Seltzer and Sherwin (1983). They divided clinically-diagnosed cases into early- and late-onset groups, using 65 years of age as the dividing point. Out of the 28 early-onset cases, six were found to be left-handed, compared to zero out of the 23 late-onset cases. In addition, they found early-onset cases to have a greater prevalence of language disorder, leading them to propose that the left hemisphere is particularly involved in these cases. Selzer and Sherwin speculated that left-handers

Table 8.1 Summary of studies comparing prevalence of left-handedness in early- and late-onset cases

Authors	Year	Prevalence of left-handedness	
		Early-onset cases	Late-onset cases
Seltzer and Sherwin	1983	6/28	0/23
Seltzer *et al.*	1984	7/31	0/32
Drexler *et al.*	1984	0/13	3/32
Loring and Largen	1985	0/13	0/24
Filley *et al.*	1986	1/23	1/18

may have increased left hemisphere vulnerability and so are particularly prone to early-onset Alzheimer's disease.

Subsequently, Seltzer *et al.* (1984) replicated the handedness findings on a further sample of early- and late-onset cases. They proposed that left-handers are particularly prone to early-onset Alzheimer's disease and so tend not to survive to late old age. Consequently, the late-onset group is left with the survivors and has a low prevalence of left-handedness.

Later studies comparing early- and late-onset cases have not, however, found a difference in handedness. The results of these studies are summarized in Table 8.1, together with the original findings of Seltzer and his colleagues. It can be seen that the original studies yielded quite different results to the later ones. A recent study by Selnes *et al.* (1988) also found no significant difference in handedness, but reported no actual data.

An important limitation of the studies of early- and late-onset cases is that they did not include normal control groups, so that it is impossible to know whether early-onset cases have an excess of left-handers, whether late-onset cases have a deficit, or both. However, other studies have used a conventional case-control approach, although without dividing cases by age of onset. The results of these studies are summarized in Table 8.2. The only study to find an association was that by de Leon *et al.* (1986) and they found left-handedness to be *less* frequent in cases than controls. The authors interpreted their results as

Table 8.2 Summary of case-control studies examining left-handedness as a risk factor

Authors	Year	Predominant age of onset	Odds ratio	Statistical significance
Soininen and Heinonen	1982	Late	?	No
Amaducci *et al.*	1986	Early	1.67* (vs. hospital controls)	No
			1.33* (vs. community controls)	No
de Leon *et al.*	1986	Mixed	0.22	Yes
Chandra *et al.*	1987a	Late	1.00	No
Becker *et al.*	1988	Mixed	0.17	No
Broe *et al.*	1990	Late	0.55	No

* Ambidextrous included with left-handers.

supporting those of Seltzer and colleagues on the grounds that their cases were mainly late-onset. However, the cases ranged in age from 60 to 80, so some must have been of early-onset. The case-control study of Chandra *et al.* (1987a) involved only late-onset cases, but did not find fewer left-handers amongst cases, nor did the study by Broe *et al.* (1990) with a group of predominantly late onset.

Given that three studies have found some association with handedness, this factor deserves further investigation. However, at this stage the evidence is too mixed to draw even tentative conclusions about possible associations or lack of them.

8.2.4 Family history of Alzheimer's disease

A family history of Alzheimer's disease is probably the most important risk factor apart from old age. However, the study of this risk factor presents particular difficulties because of the nature of Alzheimer's disease as a disorder of ageing. Studies of family history are essentially restricted to parents and siblings because children have not reached the

Table 8.3 Case-control studies of family history of dementia as a risk factor

Authors	Year	Predominant age of case onset	Odds ratio	Statistical significance
Soininen and Heinonen	1982	Late	9.90*	Yes
Pinessi *et al.*	1983	Late	?	No
Heyman *et al.*	1984	Early	7.74	Yes
Barclay *et al.*	1985c	Mixed	9.52	Yes
Amaducci *et al.*	1986	Early	6.67 (vs. hospital controls)	Yes
			3.44 (vs. community controls)	Yes
Chandra *et al.*	1987a	Late	1.00*	No
Ferini-Strambi *et al.*	1987	Early	> 1	No
Graves *et al.*	1987	?	2.1	Yes
Shalat *et al.*	1987	Early	8.6	Yes
		Late	2.3	No
Katzman *et al.*	1989	Late	0.77	No
Hofman *et al.*	1989a	Early	4.3*	Yes
Broe *et al.*	1990	Late	3.64*	Yes

* First-degree relatives only.

period of risk. Even with siblings and parents, many relatives will die before reaching late old age, forcing the assessment of familial disease to be based on few relatives. Parents present the greatest problem because they will generally have died years before, when little was known about Alzheimer's disease. Clinical diagnosis of Alzheimer's disease has a certain degree of inaccuracy in the living patient, so retrospective diagnoses must be even more inaccurate. For this reason, many studies of family history restrict their enquiry to the dementia syndrome, without attempting retrospective diagnosis of Alzheimer's disease specifically.

The ideal method of studying the effects of family history is to investigate an unbiased series of cases selected from a general population survey. However, the only such study is Åkesson's (1969) survey of dementia on the west coast of Sweden. Ideally, family history should be studied in incident cases, but Åkesson mixed both prevalent and incident cases in his study. In the families of these cases, he found the cumulative risk to age 80+ to be much higher in siblings (31%) and parents (23%) than for the rest of the population (4%).

Many case-control studies have examined family history of dementia using cases selected through clinics. These studies are summarized in Table 8.3. Overall, the studies support an association between Alzheimer's disease and a family history of dementia, with odds ratios ranging from 0.77 to 9.90. Statistically significant associations were found in eight of the twelve studies. Mortimer (1989) has carried out a meta-analysis of data from seven case-control studies reporting on family history of dementia and found a pooled odds ratio of 3.96 which was highly statistically significant.

Age of case onset seems to be an important moderating variable as far as family history is concerned. In case-control studies dealing predominantly with early-onset Alzheimer's disease (ages under 70), the associations are consistently positive and mostly statistically significant. However, with late-onset Alzheimer's disease the associations tend to be smaller and generally non-significant. Family history studies have also implicated age-of-onset as a critical variable. Perhaps the most thorough exploration of the issue is Heston's (1981) study of family history in 125 autopsy-proven cases of Alzheimer's disease. He divided cases according to onset before or after 70 years and found family history to be much stronger in the early-onset group. The risk to siblings of late-onset cases hardly differed from the general population. At the other extreme, the risk to siblings of early-onset cases who also had an affected parent approached 50%, consistent with autosomal dominant inheritance.

More recently, Thal *et al.* (1988) studied family history in a large sample of clinically-diagnosed cases and found that almost 50% of cases with onset under 55 years of age had a positive family history, compared to only 25% of those with onsets over 70 years of age. Results implicating the importance of age-of-onset also came from a re-analysis by Wright and Whalley (1984) of the classic family history studies of Sjögren *et al*. (1952) and Larsson *et al* (1963) in Sweden. Sjögren *et al*. studied the families of early-onset cases, allowing Wright and Whalley (1984) to estimate heritability for early- and late-onset disease in relatives. Heritability was found to be higher for early-onset disease in relatives (0.89) than for late-onset disease (0.44). By contrast, Larsson *et al*. (1963) studied late-onset cases. Heritability calculated from their data also gave a higher value for early-onset disease in relatives (0.83) compared to late-onset disease (0.62).

A relationship between age-of-onset and family history has not, however, been consistently found. Family history studies by Heyman *et al*. (1983), Chui *et al*. (1985) and Fitch *et al*. (1988) have found no effect of age-of-onset. The discrepancy in results is difficult to account for, but the negative studies drew on clinic cases whereas the positive ones used autopsied patients or those admitted to mental hospitals. Biases in selection into the studies could be an important factor. What is needed is a study of family history in a representative sample of cases. The only population-based study of family history (Åkesson, 1969) did not examine the effect of age-of-onset.

If age-of-onset has a critical moderating effect on the importance of family history as a risk factor, then this raises the question of whether early- and late-onset forms are in fact separate entities. A critical test of this possibility is to see whether relatives of early-onset cases are at increased risk of late-onset Alzheimer's disease, and vice versa. If there are two separate disorders, then having a relative affected by one of them should not increase risk for the other. Supporting evidence for two separate disorders comes from Larsson *et al*'s (1963) study of senile dementia. They claimed that Alzheimer's disease was completely absent in the families of their senile dementia cases. However, as Wright and Whalley (1984) have pointed out, the distinction between senile dementia and Alzheimer's disease was made on clinical grounds which no longer seem valid. If age-of-onset alone is used to separate cases into subgroups, then the senile dementia cases did have relatives with onsets before 65 years. In fact, relatives of these cases had 10–20 times higher risk of pre-senile Alzheimer's disease than the general population. In a similar vein, Constantinidis (1978) found that early- and late-onset cases occurred in the same families, with relatives of late-onset cases having greater risk of early-onset disease, and vice versa. Nevertheless, there may be some tendency for age-of-onset to be correlated in affected relatives. Heston (1981) found a correlation of 0.31 between age-of-onset in his cases and their affected siblings, and 0.47 between cases and their affected parents. Despite this correlation, relatives tended to have an older age-of-onset than the cases studied, averaging 4.8 years older in this study.

Besides age-of-onset, the major variable claimed to moderate the effects of family history is the presence of 'cortical' dysfunctions, in particular aphasia and apraxia. Breitner and Folstein observed that Alzheimer patients with aphasia and apraxia are more likely to have a positive family history than those without (Folstein and Breitner, 1981; Breitner and Folstein, 1984). They estimated lifetime risk up to age 90 for first-degree relatives and found that this exceeded 50% for the group with aphasia and apraxia, consistent with autosomal dominant inheritance. Since patients with aphasia and apraxia made up the majority of the Alzheimer cases investigated by Breitner and Folstein, they hypothesized that this autosomal dominant form of the disease is quite common. Later, Breitner *et al.* (1986) developed a statistical model for the genetics of the autosomal dominant disease. However, subsequent attempts to find an association of aphasia and apraxia with family history have been unsuccessful. In fact, Knesevich *et al.* (1985) found exactly the opposite, with non-aphasic cases more likely to have a positive family history. This study differed from the work of Breitner and Folstein (1984) in that all the patients were at the same stage of severity. In the earlier work, the aphasic/apraxic patients tended to be more advanced than the other patients. In other research on this issue, Chui *et al.* (1985) found a non-significant tendency for patients with agraphia or aphasia to have more affect family members, while Heyman *et al.* (1983) found no relationship between aphasia and familial disease.

While there is clearly some association between family history of dementia and risk for Alzheimer's disease, there is little agreement on the mechanism of the association. Many have hypothesized simple genetic mechanisms. These theories are discussed in the next chapter. However, environmental exposures in common with relatives might also explain familial effects. Genetic factors cannot, in themselves, provide a complete account because there are now numerous reports of monozygotic twins discordant for Alzheimer's disease (Nee *et al.*, 1987; Creasey *et al.*, 1989). Environmental factors must be responsible for these discordances.

8.2.5 Dementia in spouses

While dementia in first-degree relatives can be interpreted in either genetic or environmental terms, dementia in spouses provides a clear test of the environmental account. If spouses have a high incidence of dementia, then shared adult environment must be responsible. Otherwise, genetic factors or childhood environmental factors are implicated.

Relatively few studies have examined dementia in spouses of Alzheimer's disease cases, perhaps because spouses often serve as informants and hence must not be themselves dementing. Larsson *et al.* (1963), in their classic study of late-onset Alzheimer's disease in Sweden, found that spouses had no greater risk of being affected than the general population, unlike biological relatives. More recent family history studies by Breitner and Folstein (1984), Mohs *et al.* (1987) and Huff *et al.* (1988) have found results consistent with Larsson *et al.* (1963). The cumulative incidence of Alzheimer's disease in spouses was found to be similar to that in relatives of controls. These results do not give any support to the view that shared adult environment is responsible for the increased risk in biological relatives.

8.2.6 Family history of Down's syndrome

Heston (1981) was the first to report an increased risk for Down's syndrome in the families of Alzheimer's disease cases. He found a rate of 1 for every 240 births, against the expected 1 in 700 in the general population. Most of the relatives affected by Down's were quite distant, making a simple genetic interpretation difficult. However, Heston argued that most first-degree relatives were born before 1900 and that Down's was often not diagnosed at that time. Therefore, there may have been affected first-degree relatives not known to his study. Heston also found that the risk of relatives being affected by Down's varied with age of case onset. For Alzheimer's cases with onset before age 50, the risk was 1 in 100, but this diminished to the level found for the general population with the relatives of the oldest cases.

Heston's (1981) finding has been replicated in two case-control studies. In a study of early-onset cases, Heyman *et al.* (1984) found mental retardation (including Down's) to occur in the relatives of 15% of the cases compared to only 4% of the controls. The odds ratio of 4.0 was statistically significant. Broe *et al.* (1990) found Down's in first-degree relatives for 3% of their cases, but none of the controls. This yielded a significant odds ratio of 9.0. In contrast to the earlier positive studies, this one was with a predominantly late-onset group.

Three other case-control studies have produced negative results (Barclay *et al.*, 1985c; Amaducci *et al.*, 1986; Chandra *et al.*, 1987a). However, each of these studies failed to find any instances of Down's in the families of controls. Because the frequency of Down's in control family members was so low, these studies did not provide a strong test of whether an association exists. Interestingly, Down's was found in families of cases in each study: for two out of 259 cases in the Barclay *et al.* (1985c) study, for one out of 114 in the Amaducci *et al.* (1986) study and two out of 64 in the Chandra *et al.* (1987a) study.

In a family pedigree study, Whalley *et al.* (1982) also had difficulty evaluating this association because of the rarity of Down's in families. They found no instances of Down's in the first-degree relatives of their autopsy-proven Alzheimer cases. However, they did not personally interview the families, but relied on available data from a cytogenetics unit. Therefore, some Down's cases may have been missed. Furthermore, with only 329 siblings and children in these families, and an expected rate of 1/700 in the general population, a zero occurrence might be expected. Another family history study by Fitch *et al.* (1988) also looked for Down's in families. They found three cases but, because they did not report the number of relatives studied, it is impossible to calculate a rate. However, all three cases occurred in relatives of 52 'non-familial' cases, while no instances of Down's were found in relatives of 39 'familial' cases (where at least one other family member was affected by Alzheimer's disease). A genetic hypothesis would have predicted the opposite pattern. Martin *et al.* (1988) and Huff *et al.* (1988) have also investigated Down's as part of family history studies of Alzheimer's disease. Both studies found no instances of Down's syndrome in either Alzheimer or control families.

While several studies have investigated the occurrence of Down's syndrome in relatives of Alzheimer's disease cases, the reverse association has received little attention. The only study of the subject was carried out in Ireland by Yatham *et al.* (1988). They sent letters to the parents or guardians of all Down's cases in South Dublin asking about signs of Alzheimer's disease in first- and second-degree relatives. Amongst those responding to the questionnaire, 9% of families were found to have a relative with signs suggestive of Alzheimer's disease. The number with pre-senile Alzheimer's disease was found to exceed expectation based on published prevalence figures, but there was no excess of senile cases. While this study supports familial association between Down's and pre-senile Alzheimer's disease, the results need to be treated with caution because only 52% of families responded to the questionnaire. If the responders were more likely to have cases of Alzheimer's disease in their families, then the results would be biased in favour of the hypothesis.

Taking all of the evidence together, there is reason to suspect a possible link between Alzheimer's disease and Down's syndrome in relatives. However, the incidence of Down's syndrome is so low in the general population, that studies with very large samples are needed to adequately assess whether there is an excess in relatives of Alzheimer's disease cases.

8.2.7 Family history of haematological malignancies

A link with family history of haematological malignancies was first proposed by Heston (1981). He was led to investigate this association because of previous work showing that such malignancies are common in Down's syndrome and in the families of Down's cases. In a family history study of autopsy-proven Alzheimer's disease cases, Heston found that haematological malignancies were 4.61 times more common in first-degree relatives of cases than in relatives of controls. The malignancies were mostly in cells of lymphocytic tissues; lymphocytic leukaemias, multiple myeloma, Hodgkin's disease and lymphomas. With second-degree relatives the risk was greatly lessened. Even in first-degree relatives the risk was largely concentrated in those of early-onset cases. Heston favoured a genetic interpretation of these findings.

The results of Heston's study prompted a number of other investigators to study haematological malignancies in relatives. However, the results from these studies have been largely negative. A number of these studies have used a similar family history approach to Heston's. Whalley *et al.* (1982), like Heston, studied families of autopsy-proven cases. They found two instances of immunoproliferative disorders in first-degree relatives, which was little different from the three cases expected in a comparable group from the general population. As the cases investigated by Whalley *et al.* (1982) were all early-onset, the chances of detecting any association should have been good. Three other family history studies, also failed to find an increase in haemato-logical malignancies (Breitner and Folstein, 1984; Fitch *et al.*, 1988; Huff *et al.*, 1988). These differed from Heston's (1981) work in using clinically-diagnosed cases. Breitner and Folstein's (1984) study also involved cases of late-onset, so little association might be expected. The only family history study to support an association is that by Martin *et al.* (1988). They found three instances of haematological malignancies in first-degree relatives of 22 cases, but none in relatives of 24 controls. This difference was statistically significant. Most of the Alzheimer cases in this study were early-onset, but there were late-onset ones too.

Four case-control studies have also examined family history of haemoto-logical malignancies as a risk factor. Heyman *et al.* (1984) studied early-onset cases, but found an odds ratio of only 1.1 for leukaemia and haematological malignancies in relatives. Amaducci *et al.* (1986) also studied mainly early-onset cases and looked at leukaemia in their first-degree relatives. They found an odds ratio of only 0.3 for hospital controls, and only 0.5 for community controls, indicating that cases were *less* likely to have had a family history of leukaemia. Chandra *et al.* (1987a) studied late-onset cases and found an odds ratio of 0.3 for haematological malignancies in first-degree relatives, again indicating a lower risk for a family history in cases. Finally, Broe *et al.* (1990) found a non-significant odds ratio of 3.00, with mainly late-onset cases.

In summary, the evidence on family history of haematological malig-nancies is generally negative apart from Heston's (1981) original study reporting an association and the recent replication by Martin *et al.* (1988). If any association does exist it must be a weak one.

8.3 BIRTH FACTORS AND FERTILITY

8.3.1 Parental age

Because the major risk factor for Down's syndrome is advanced maternal age, researchers have been led to look for a similar association with Alzheimer's disease. The issue was first investigated by Åkesson (1969) as part of his community survey of prevalence and incidence in western Sweden. He found no difference between his cases and controls from the same population. However, interest in maternal age was re-awakened when Cohen *et al.* (1982) reported that maternal age was higher in a clinic series than in a randomly selected series of birth records from the

Table 8.4 Summary of studies evaluating maternal age as a risk factor

Authors	Year	Mean maternal age for cases	Mean maternal age for controls	Statistical significance
Åkesson	1969	33.0	31.7	No
Cohen *et al.*	1982	35.5*	27.0*	Yes
Whalley *et al.*	1982	30.6	28.6	Yes
Knesevich *et al.*	1982	27.7 (clinically diagnosed) 28.0 (autopsy diagnosed)	30.4	No
Corkin *et al.*	1983	27.7	27.4	No
Heyman *et al.*	1983	28.6	28.4	No
English and Cohen	1985	29.1†	28.8†	No
White *et al.*	1986	29.1	27.5	No
Urakami *et al.*	1988	26.6	24.1	Yes
De Braekeleer *et al.*	1988	29.4	29.1–31.5	No‡
Katzman *et al.*	1989	25.0	26.0	No
Hofman *et al.*	1989b	28.6	29.3	No
Jouan-Flahault *et al.*	1989	28.5	28.2	No

* Median ages.
† Means estimated from grouped frequency distribution.
‡ Maternal age for cases was significantly lower compared to one of eight control groups studied.

same era. Since then, a number of others have looked at maternal age in clinic series. Those studies which reported mean maternal ages are summarized in Table 8.4. It can be seen that three of the 13 studies found a significantly higher mean maternal age in cases. There was also one significant result in the opposite direction (De Braekeleer *et al.*, 1988), but this study involved comparing cases to eight different control groups, only one of which gave the significant result. When the direction of the means is examined in Table 8.4, it is found that cases have higher mean maternal ages in nine of the 13 studies.

In addition to the above studies, there are two others which investigated maternal age, but reported odds ratios rather than means. Amaducci *et al.* (1986) calculated the odds ratio for the mother to be aged 40+ at delivery. A statistically significant odds ratio of 4.67 was found comparing cases to community controls, but a non-significant value of 2.50 comparing them to hospital controls. Dewey *et al.* (1988) studied maternal age in a community survey of dementia (not Alzheimer's disease specifically). They grouped maternal age into several bands, and found an odds ratio of 1.01, indicating no difference.

Taking all the results together, the bulk of the evidence has been negative. However, there have been four statistically significant results out of 15 studies, which is more than expected by chance, and the trend is for the maternal age of cases to be higher in 11 of these studies. If maternal age is a true risk factor for Alzheimer's disease the size of the effect must be very small and by no means comparable to that found with Down's syndrome.

Such a small effect could arise if late maternal age were a risk factor for only a subgroup of cases. Studies primarily involving this subgroup

Table 8.5 Summary of studies evaluating paternal age as a risk factor

Authors	Year	Mean paternal age for cases	Mean paternal age for controls	Statistical significance
Whalley *et al.*	1982	33.2	30.8	Yes
Corkin *et al.*	1983	30.8	29.4	No
Heyman *et al.*	1983	33.3	31.9	No
White *et al.*	1986	34.2	32.9	No
Urakami *et al.*	1988	31.4	27.2	Yes
De Braekeleer *et al.*	1988	32.6	32.2–34.9	No*
Hofman *et al.*	1989b	30.7	32.2	No
Jouan-Flahault *et al.*	1989	31.6	33.0	No

* Paternal age for cases was significantly *lower* compared to one of eight control groups studied.

would show the maternal age effect, whereas studies with fewer cases from the subgroup would not. Schoenberg *et al.* (1988) have suggested that familial and sporadic cases may differ in the importance of maternal age as a risk factor. Using data from Amaducci *et al.* (1986), they divided the cases into two groups according to whether or not at least one first-degree relative was affected by Alzheimer's disease. With the sporadic cases, maternal age over 40 years was significantly more common compared to both hospital and community controls (odds ratios of 4.5 and 6.0). However, there was no significant difference with familial cases (odds ratios of 0.5 and 2.0). Later, Hofman *et al.* (1989b) tried unsuccessfully to replicate this finding. They found an odds ratio of only 0.9 for maternal age of more than 40 years in sporadic cases.

Paternal age has received far less attention than maternal age. The studies reporting mean paternal ages are summarized in Table 8.5. In addition, there are the studies which calculated odds ratios. The case-control study by Amaducci *et al.* (1986) looked at the frequency of having a father aged 44+ at birth. They found an odds ratio of 0.60 using hospital controls and 4.50 using community controls. Dewey *et al.*'s (1988) study found an odds ratio of 1.04 for their grouping of paternal age. Taking all the studies together, only two have found a significantly increased paternal age (Whalley *et al.*, 1982; Urakami *et al.*, 1988), while the others have found small and inconsistent differences.

8.3.2 Birth order

The number of previous births from the parents may be the crucial variable rather than high parental age, as the two factors tend to correlate. Several studies have examined birth order but, because of the diverse methods of reporting such effects, it is impossible to compare directly the results obtained. However, none of the studies investigating birth order has yielded statistically significant results (Larsson *et al.*, 1963; Åkesson, 1969; Amaducci *et al.*, 1982; Knesevich *et al.*, 1982; Whalley *et al.*, 1982; White *et al.*, 1986; Chandra *et al.*, 1987a; De Braekeleer *et al.*, 1988).

8.3.3 Fertility

Fertility of Alzheimer's disease cases (i.e. number of offspring) has been reported in several studies. The results of these studies seem to vary with the sex of the cases. Table 8.6 shows the results with samples which are entirely or predominantly female. These studies tend to show lower fertility in female cases. The only exception to this general finding is the study by Larsson *et al.* (1963) of patients from Stockholm mental hospitals. These cases had greater fertility than the total Stockholm

Table 8.6 Fertility in females with Alzheimer's disease

Authors	Year	Mean number of children		Percentage of females in sample	Statistical significance
		Cases	Controls		
Larsson *et al.*	1963	1.66*	1.50 (Stockholm)*	100	?
			2.45 (Sweden)*	100	?
Whalley *et al.*	1982	1.88	2.49	100	No
Soininen and Heinonen	1982	?	?	75	No
Heyman *et al.*	1984	2.2	2.8	70	No
Coquoz	1984	1.85*	3.05*	100	?
Gaillard	1984	1.61*	2.56* (for 1931)	100	?
			2.35* (for 1945)	100	?
White *et al.*	1986	2.67	2.85	100	No

* Includes married women only.

population from the same birth cohort, but less than the total Swedish birth cohort. Because of migration of cases from the rest of Sweden to Stockholm, it is unclear which of these provided the more appropriate comparison.

Less information is available on fertility in male cases. Table 8.7 summarizes two studies of the issue. In the study by White *et al.* (1986), male cases had significantly greater fertility than controls. In the Larsson *et al.* (1963) study, however, fertility could be seen as higher or lower depending on whether Stockholm or the rest of Sweden was used for comparison purposes.

Table 8.7 Fertility in males with Alzheimer's disease

Authors	Year	Mean number of children		Percentage of females in sample	Statistical significance
		Cases	Controls		
Larsson *et al.*	1963	2.45*	2.10 (Stockholm)*	100	?
			3.10 (Sweden)*	100	?
White *et al.*	1986	3.29	2.37	100	Yes

* Includes married men only.

While it is possible that Alzheimer's disease is associated with reduced fertility in females, case selection factors could also be responsible.
Women with few or no offspring might be more likely to come to the
attention of specialist clinics or be hospitalized because there is nobody
available to care for them in the community. Studies of fertility in unselected general population samples are needed to investigate the issue
properly. While no such studies are available specifically on Alzheimer's
disease, Kay *et al.* (1964b) have reported on fertility in cases of dementia
detected as part of a community survey. They found that demented
males had more children than either normals or those with functional
psychiatric disorders, and the difference was statistically significant. For
females, a similar trend was observed, but the difference was not
statistically significant. However, this study excluded institutionalized
cases, so there may have been an offsetting lower fertility in this group
Further investigation of fertility in general population samples is war-
ranted.

8.4 OCCUPATIONAL AND RECREATIONAL EXPOSURES

Particular occupations or recreational pursuits could be associated with
exposures to toxins or infectious agents. The possibility of such exposures
has been examined in a number of case-control studies.

8.4.1 Occupational exposures

The most thorough coverage of occupational exposures was in the case-
control study by French *et al.* (1985). This study looked at exposure to
textiles, pesticides, anaesthetic gases, X-rays, drugs, dry-cleaning solu-
tions, solvents, extreme temperatures, carbon monoxide, plastics, vibratory tools, metals, cleaning compounds and laboratory chemicals. For
none of these exposures was the odds ratio statistically significant.
Similar conclusions were reached in other case-control studies. Heyman
et al. (1984) stated that none of their patients or controls had occupations
involving considerable exposure to toxic chemicals or heavy metals.
Chandra *et al.* (1987a) found only 4.7% of their cases and 1.6% of
controls had occupations involving possible exposures to toxic or
infectious agents, while Barclay *et al.* (1985c) found job-related toxic
exposures in only 1.5% of cases and 0.9% of controls. Shalat *et al.* (1988)
specifically investigated exposure to organic solvents and lead as risk
factors, but found very similar rates of exposure in both cases and
controls.

While the results of case-control studies are consistently negative, this
should not be taken to mean that occupational exposures are not
involved in Alzheimer's disease. The frequency of any particular occu-

pational exposure is so low that few, if any, instances may turn up in a case-control study. These studies are only useful in detecting the effects of relatively common exposures. Focused studies of particular occupational groups are needed to research the issue adequately.

The only body of research on dementia in particular occupational groups deals with the so-called 'painter's syndrome'. Research on dementia in painters has been confined to the Scandinavian countries, in particular Denmark, where the syndrome has received wide attention. Axelson *et al.* (1976), in Sweden, carried out a case-control study of neuropsychiatric disorders in workers exposed to solvents, including painters, varnishers and carpet layers. From their data, an odds ratio of 2.51 for dementia can be calculated. Similarly, in a cohort study of Danish painters, Mikkelsen (1980) reported a relative risk of approximately 2 for disability pension or death due to dementia. In a subsequent cohort study, Mikkelsen *et al.* (1988) were able to carry out a neuropsychological assessment of their subjects. This study found a dose–response effect, with an odds ratio of close to 1.0 for low exposure to solvents, rising to an odds ratio of around 5.0 for high exposure. In a community study of dementia prevalence, Nielsen *et al.* (1982) found a number of painters and estimated a relative prevalence ratio of 2, which was not statistically significant. While some studies indicate a small increase in risk for dementia amongst painters, these studies have been severely criticized by Errebo-Knudsen and Olsen (1986) who argued that there is no firm evidence to support the existence of the painter's syndrome. They believe an increased risk for painters can be accounted for by low pre-morbid intelligence, alcohol consumption, cerebrovascular disease, and that the existing studies have failed to meet basic methodological requirements such as keeping subjects blind to the purposes of the study. Whether or not the painter's syndrome exists, it is not claimed to be a progressive dementia and there is no evidence for Alzheimer neuropathology.

Other occupations to be specifically investigated are hold-labourers on fishing boats and users of vibratory tools. Jessen and Svennild (1986) found no evidence that dementia is more common in the former, while Iivanainen (1975) reported that use of vibratory tools at work was associated with diffuse cerebral atrophy. However, there was no suggestion that this atrophy was associated with the neuropathological or clinical features of Alzheimer's disease.

8.4.2 Exposure to animals

Because of the possibility that Alzheimer's disease results from an infectious agent, several case-control studies have examined exposure to animals as a possible source of infection. The results of studies which

Table 8.8 Summary of case-control studies dealing with animal exposures

Authors	Year	Odds ratio	Statistical significance
Exposure to pets			
Heyman *et al.*	1984	1.00	No
French *et al.*	1985	?	No
Amaducci *et al.*	1986	2.36 (vs. hospital controls)	Yes
		0.95 (vs. community controls)	No
Chandra *et al.*	1987a	0.94	No
Dewey *et al.**	1988	0.95	No
Exposure to wildlife (hunting, trapping)			
Heyman *et al.*	1984	0.46	No
French *et al.*	1985	?	No
Amaducci *et al.*	1986	1.00 (vs. hospital controls)	No
		1.25 (vs. community controls)	No
Chandra *et al.*	1987a	0.67	No
Exposure to livestock (or working on farm)			
Heyman *et al.*	1984	0.70	No
French *et al.*	1985	? (vs. hospital controls)	Yes (controls more exposed)
		? (vs. neighbourhood controls)	No
Amaducci *et al.*	1986	1.63 (vs. hospital controls)	No
		1.22 (vs. community controls)	No
Chandra *et al.*	1987a	1.00	No
Broe *et al.*	1990	1.40	No

* Looked at dementia syndrome, rather than Alzheimer's disease specifically.

have examined exposure to pets, wildlife or livestock are summarized in Table 8.8. The results of these studies are generally negative. Amaducci *et al.* (1986) did find exposure to pets to be more common in cases than in hospital controls, but this was not replicated with community controls. Also, French *et al.* (1985) found that cases had been less exposed to livestock than hospital controls, who were more likely to come from rural areas, but this could not be replicated with neighbourhood controls. Taking the findings as a whole, the odds ratios are generally low and cluster around 1.0, leading to the conclusion that there is unlikely to be an association with animal exposures.

8.4.3 Travel in the South Pacific

The native people of Guam and certain other regions of the Pacific are known to have a high incidence of a dementing disease with neuropathological similarities to Alzheimer's disease. It is possible that travellers to these regions are exposed to some risk factor for this dementia. Consequently, Heyman *et al.* (1984) assessed whether their American cases were more likely to have travelled to the South Pacific, particularly during World War II. They found that 12.5% of their cases had travelled to the Orient or South Pacific compared with 3.8% of controls, but the difference was not statistically significant. Chandra *et al.* (1987a) also looked at travel overseas, especially to the South Pacific in their case-control study. They found an odds ratio of 0.93, indicating no relationship with this exposure.

Since these studies were published it has been suggested that the dementia found in Guam is due to consumption of the cycad seed (Spencer *et al.*, 1987). This seed contains neurotoxins which could compound the effects of age-related neuronal loss. Cycad seed consumption is a very unlikely exposure for individuals of developed countries.

8.5 PREVIOUS ILLNESS AND INJURIES

8.5.1 Head trauma

Repeated blows to the head, such as occur in boxing, are known to cause dementia sometimes. Corsellis (1978) reported that this dementia pugilistica is associated with large numbers of neurofibrillary tangles, but not with senile plaques. Dementia pugilistica is therefore related to Alzheimer's disease, but is not identical to it. However, there are a number of case reports in the literature of single major blows to the head being followed by dementia of the Alzheimer type. Ruddelli *et al* (1982) have reported such a case and summarized earlier reports of six similar cases. In these cases, a progressive dementia started 0–11 years after a single incident of head trauma and autopsy showed the presence of both plaques and tangles. In most of these cases, the dementia began when the patient was aged over 50, so it is possible that Alzheimer's disease coincidentally followed head trauma. However, in the case reported by Rudelli *et al.* (1982) the incident of head trauma was at age 22 and the dementia began at age 30, leading to death at age 37. The very young age of this case makes coincidental Alzheimer's disease an unlikely explanation.

The possibility that head trauma is a risk factor for Alzheimer's disease has been investigated in a number of case-control studies. Generally, head trauma is defined in these studies as an injury to the head resulting in loss of consciousness. The results of the studies are summarized in Table 8.9. Of the twelve studies, only three have yielded statistically significant associations, and for one of these three studies a

Table 8.9 Summary of case-control studies examining head trauma as a risk factor

Authors	Year	Odds ratio	Statistical significance
Soininen and Heinonen	1982	0.63	No
Heyman *et al.*	1984	5.31	Yes
Mortimer *et al.*	1985a	4.50 (vs. hospital controls)	Yes
		2.80 (vs. neighbourhood controls)	No
Barclay *et al.*	1986c	0.49	No
Amaducci *et al.*	1986	3.50 (vs. hospital controls)	No
		2.00 (vs. community controls)	No
Chandra *et al.*	1987a	6.00	No
Ferini-Strambi *et al.*	1987	> 1	No
Graves *et al.*	1987	2.8	Yes
Shalat *et al.*	1987	2.4	No
Katzman *et al.*	1989	0.93	No
Van Duijn *et al.*	1989	1.4	No
Broe *et al.*	1990	1.33	No

significant result was found using hospital controls but not using neighbourhood controls. However, odds ratios from the other studies are generally greater than 1.0, and three statistically significant results exceeds the expectation from chance. The negative result from the study of Barclay *et al.* (1985c) merits special discussion. In this study, only a third of the cases were males, compared to 62% of the controls. Mortimer *et al.* (1985b) have pointed out that the incidence of head trauma is 2–3 times higher in males than in females. Therefore, the lower incidence of head trauma which Barclay *et al.* (1985) found in cases may be due to the failure to match for sex. Mortimer (1989) has carried out a meta-analysis of data from eight of the earlier case-control studies reporting on head trauma (Barclay *et al.*, 1985c, was excluded) and found a pooled odds ratio of 2.77, which was highly statistically significant.

In their case-control study, Van Duijn *et al.* (1989) considered the possibility that head trauma could be a risk factor for only a subgroup of cases. They subdivided their cases into familial and sporadic groups, where a familial case was defined as having at least one affected first-degree relative. Head trauma emerged as a significant risk factor for the sporadic cases (odds ratio of 2.6), but not for the familial ones (odds ratio of 0.7). When both groups were combined, the overall association was small and non-significant. Other studies have not subdivided cases in this way, but it obviously merits attempts at replication.

In addition to the above case-control studies, Sulkava *et al.* (1985b) have reported on head trauma in clinically-diagnosed cases of Alzheimer's and vascular dementia. They found a history of head trauma in 6.1% of the Alzheimer cases compared to 9.9% of vascular cases. Sulkava *et al.* (1985b) argued from this result that head trauma is not a risk factor for Alzheimer's disease. However, without a normal control group it is impossible to draw any firm conclusions. It could be that head trauma is a risk factor for both Alzheimer and vascular dementias, thus producing no difference between them.

In contrast to the above studies based on clinical series, D'Alessandro *et al.* (1988) looked at the role of head trauma in cases detected as part of a field study of prevalence. Previous head trauma was found in none of the cases, compared to 3% of healthy subjects. However, since only 11 cases of Alzheimer's disease were studied, this negative result cannot be given much weight.

Case-control studies indicate that head trauma could be a genuine risk factor. It is also a theoretically plausible risk factor because it is easy to imagine head trauma disrupting neural processes and precipitating the onset of a neurological disease. However, this theoretical plausibility is also a reason for caution. Case-control studies rely on retrospective reports from relatives about past incidents of head trauma. Because of the plausibility, incidents of head trauma may be recalled better by relatives of cases than by relatives of controls.

The way to overcome recall bias is to use prospective studies in which head trauma is ascertained before the onset of Alzheimer's disease. This has been done in two studies. Lewin *et al.* (1979) followed up 291 consecutive cases admitted to hospital for head injuries and who had been unconscious for a week or more. The follow-up period varied from 10 to 24 years. Progressive dementia was found in 11% at follow-up, which seems a high rate for a group which was predominantly young or middle-aged. However, no control group was used and the type of dementing disorder was not ascertained. In the other prospective study, Chandra *et al.* (1987b) ascertained Alzheimer's disease and head trauma with loss of consciousness using medical records for the whole community of Rochester in Minnesota. They compared 296 cases of Alzheimer's disease with matched community controls. The odds ratio for exposure to head trauma was only 1.2 and not statistically significant.

Further prospective studies are needed before any definitive conclusion can be reached about head trauma. However, it must be regarded as a possible risk factor for Alzheimer's disease.

8.5.2 Thyroid disease

A statistically significant association between Alzheimer's disease and a history of thyroid disease was noted in the case-control study of Heyman *et al.* (1984). No particular type of thyroid disease predominated.

Heyman *et al.* thought the association was unlikely to be a direct effect of thyroid activity on cognitive function, but rather reflected an association with autoimmune disorder. Since then, nine other case-control studies have also investigated the relationship, yielding the results shown in Table 8.10. Only one of the later studies found a statistically significant association (Amaducci *et al.*, 1986) and this was in the reverse direction,

Table 8.10   Summary of case-control studies on history of thyroid disease as a risk factor

Authors	Year	Odds ratio		Statistical significance
Heyman *et al.*	1984	3.50		Yes
Barclay *et al.*	1985c	∞*		No
French *et al.*	1985	1.67		No
Small *et al.*	1985	0.81		No
Amaducci *et al.*	1986	2.33	(vs. hospital controls)	No
		0.20	(vs. community controls)	Yes
Chandra *et al.*	1987a	0.30		No
Ferini-Strambi *et al.*	1987	> 1		No
Shalat *et al.*	1987	5.20		No
Katzman *et al.*	1989	0.67		No
Broe *et al.*	1990	1.00		No

* No controls with history of thyroid disease.

with community controls having more thyroid disease than cases. Given that only six of the 11 odds ratios in the table are greater than 1.0, and that the two statistically significant associations are in opposite directions, there is unlikely to be any but a weak association between Alzheimer's disease and a history of thyroid disease. A meta-analysis of data from seven studies by Mortimer (1989) yielded a pooled odds ratio of 1.53 which was not statistically significant.

8.5.3 Diabetes

Diabetes has been examined as a risk factor in eight studies, as shown in Table 8.11. In none of these has a statistically significant association emerged, and the odds ratios reported in these studies cluster around 1.0. Therefore, it is unlikely that diabetes has an association with Alzheimer's disease.

Table 8.11 Summary of case-control studies examining diabetes as a risk factor

Authors	Year	Odds ratio	Statistical significance
Soininen and Heinonen	1982	?	No
Pinessi *et al.*	1983	?	No
Heyman *et al.*	1984	0.84	No
French *et al.*	1985	0.78	No
Amaducci *et al.*	1986	0.71 (vs. hospital controls)	No
		1.00 (vs. community controls)	No
Shalat *et al.*	1987	1.60	No
Katzman *et al.*	1989	0.53	No
Broe *et al.*	1990	0.56	No

8.5.4 Meningitis and encephalitis

Case-control studies have failed to detect any associations of meningitis or encephalitis with Alzheimer's disease. Non-significant results have been noted by Soininen and Heinonen (1982) for central nervous system infections generally and by Barclay *et al.* (1985c) for meningitis. Shalat *et al.* (1987) reported a non-significant odds ratio of 3.2 for meningitis, French *et al.* (1985) reported an odds ratio of 2.00 for meningitis and encephalitis, while Broe *et al.* (1990) found an odds ratio of only 0.50 for exposure to these two diseases. Heyman *et al.* (1984) and Amaducci *et al.* (1986) found the diseases to be so rare that no meaningful conclusions could be drawn.

8.5.5 Herpes infection

Infection by herpes zoster (shingles) has been assessed as a potential risk factor in the case-control studies listed in Table 8.12. None of these studies has found a statistically significant effect and the reported odds ratios cluster around 1.0, making it unlikely that any association exists.

Herpes simplex infection (cold sores, genital herpes) has received less attention in case-control studies. Only two studies have assessed it as a potential risk factor. Bharucha *et al.* (1983) failed to find a significant association, while the study of Amaducci *et al.* (1986) yielded more complex results – genital herpes was found to be significantly more common in cases compared to community controls, but this could not be replicated with hospital controls. No association was found with labial herpes, using either control group.

Table 8.12 Summary of case-control studies examining herpes zoster (shingles) as a risk factor

Authors	Year	Odds ratio	Statistical significance
Bharucha *et al.*	1983	≈ 4.00	No
Heyman *et al.*	1984	3.33	No
Barclay *et al.*	1985c	0.00*	No
French *et al.*	1985	0.75	No
Amaducci *et al.*	1986	0.62 (vs. hospital controls)	No
		1.25 (vs. community controls)	No
Chandra *et al.*	1987a	1.30	No
Broe *et al.*	1990	0.74	No

* 0 cases and 1 control exposed.

Several immunological studies have also investigated the possibility of an association. Herpes simplex viral genome has been reported in the brain tissue of two patients with Alzheimer's disease by Sequiera *et al.* (1979), suggesting a possible association. However, this study did not include normal control brains, so the findings cannot be given too much weight. A similar study by Middleton *et al.* (1980) of five demented individuals found no evidence of infection in any case. Whalley *et al.* (1980) examined antibodies to herpes simplex and other viruses in early-onset Alzheimer cases, but found no infection common to all cases. However, this study did not use a control group. Lycke *et al.* (1974) did compare a group of demented patients with controls and found a significantly higher incidence of herpes simplex antibodies in the patients; but their controls were considerably younger than the demented patients. Only a study by Mann *et al.* (1981) has used appropriate controls. They studied necropsy brain tissue from 12 Alzheimer's disease cases and biopsy tissue from ten cases, and compared them to appropriate controls. Evidence of herpes simplex infection was found in only one biopsied Alzheimer case and this was confined to a very small brain area. Overall, adequately controlled immunological studies have not established an association between Alzheimer's disease and herpes simplex virus infection.

8.5.6 Heart disease

Soininen and Heinonen (1982) have reported that Alzheimer cases suffer less often from angina pectoris and cardiac arrhythmias, while French *et al.* (1985) have reported significantly less 'heart disease other than heart attack and angina' in cases. Other studies have failed to find significant differences in heart disease (Bharucha *et al.*, 1983; Heyman *et al.*, 1984; Barclay *et al.*, 1985c; Shalat *et al.*, 1987; Katzman *et al.*, 1989; Broe *et al.*, 1990), but there has been a tendency towards less heart disease in cases than controls. These differences may be artefacts of subject selection procedures. If the Ischemic Score (see Chapter 2) is used for clinical diagnosis of Alzheimer's disease, cases with heart disease may tend to be eliminated. Furthermore, certain commonly used control groups may be biased towards subjects with heart disease. For example, French *et al.* (1985) used hospital controls and hospital patients have a higher rate of heart disease.

Because of artefacts associated with the selection of cases or controls, it is impossible to draw any conclusions from existing case-control studies evaluating heart disease as a risk factor.

8.5.7 Stomach ulcer

Stomach ulcers could possibly be associated with Alzheimer's disease because they are often treated with aluminium-containing antacids and aluminium is a constituent of the cores of senile plaques. However, in five case-control studies, no significant association has been observed (Bharucha *et al.*, 1983; Heyman *et al.*, 1984; Barclay *et al.*, 1985c; French *et al.*, 1985; Katzman *et al.*, 1989; Broe *et al.*, 1990). In fact, in the four studies where odds ratios were reported, they were all less than 1.0, providing strong support for the conclusion that stomach ulcers are not a risk factor.

8.5.8 Kidney disease

Soininen and Heinonen (1982) have reported that chronic pyelonephritis was significantly more common in cases than controls. However, this may have been a co-morbid factor rather than a risk factor, in that Alzheimer's disease could make a person more susceptible to kidney infection. Other case-control studies by Heyman *et al.* (1984), French *et al.* (1985) and Broe *et al.* (1990) have not found significant associations of kidney disease with Alzheimer's disease and their reported odds ratios were rather low (1.12, 0.88 and 1.15, respectively). A similarly low odds ratio (0.55) was found in Dewey *et al*'s (1988) study of the dementia syndrome.

8.5.9 Arthritis

Three case-control studies have failed to find arthritis as a statistically significant risk factor (Heyman *et al.*, 1984; Barclay *et al.*, 1985c; French *et al.*, 1985), while in another it emerged as a significant protection factor

(Broe *et al.*, 1990). The latter finding makes no theoretical sense and may be a Type I error.

8.5.10 Sleep apnoea and snoring

An association between sleep apnoea and Alzheimer's disease has been reported in several studies. Smirne *et al.* (1981), were the first to note an unusually high prevalence of sleep apnoea in Alzheimer patients, but their study had no control group. Later, Smallwood *et al.* (1983) did include controls, but found sleep apnoea to be related to old age and male gender rather than to Alzheimer's disease. However, only 15 Alzheimer patients were studied, which is quite a small sample. A larger controlled study was reported by Hoch *et al.* (1986) and also in Reynolds *et al.* (1985). They found sleep apnoea to be present in 42% of cases compared to only 5% of controls. Results consistent with these were found in a controlled study by Mant *et al.* (1988). This study dealt with the dementia syndrome, rather than specifically with Alzheimer's disease, but found disturbed breathing in 72% of demented subjects compared to 46% of controls. Other data suggest that the association with sleep apnoea may not be specific to Alzheimer's disease. Erkinjuntti *et al.* (1987c) found that sleep apnoea was more common in both Alzheimer and vascular dementia cases compared to controls.

Snoring is a correlate of sleep apnoea and has also been investigated in demented patients. Erkinjuntti *et al.* (1987a) found snoring to be twice as common in demented patients, but again there was no difference between Alzheimer and vascular patients. However, the case-control study by Broe *et al.* (1990) failed to find a significant association, with odds ratios of 0.97 for being a loud snorer in the previous 10 years, and 0.80 for being one earlier in life.

The association between sleep apnoea and Alzheimer's disease is open to a number of interpretations. Sleep apnoea could be a causal factor in Alzheimer's disease by depriving the brain of oxygen during sleep. Alternatively, sleep apnoea could be a consequence of the neural degeneration which occurs in Alzheimer's disease. A third alternative is that sleep apnoea is a consequence of the disease, but acts to accelerate the rate of cognitive decline. No one has yet suggested that sleep apnoea has a direct causal role. Mant *et al.* (1988) thought this unlikely because few of their demented subjects had a long history of snoring or other indicators of sleep apnoea. Prospective studies are needed to gain a better understanding of the direction of causality, particularly whether sleep apnoea might accelerate existing cognitive decline.

8.5.11 Allergies

Case-control studies examining allergies as a possible risk factor are

Table 8.13 Summary of case-control studies evaluating allergies as a risk factor

Authors	Year	Type of allergy	Odds ratio	Statistical significance
French *et al.*	1985	Hayfever	2.75	No
		Food allergy	1.00	No
		Drug allergy	1.20	No
		Allergic dermatitis	1.56	No
		Other allergies	0.75	No
Amaducci *et al.*	1986	Hayfever	0.78 (vs. hospital controls)	No
			1.00 (vs. community controls)	No
		Allergic dermatitis	2.18 (vs. hospital controls)	Yes
			0.79 (vs. community controls)	No
Shalat *et al.*	1987	Hayfever and other allergies	1.10	No
Broe *et al.*	1990	Hayfever and other allergies	1.11	No

summarized in Table 8.13. The only statistically significant result is from Amaducci *et al.* (1986) with allergic dermatitis. This result was found with hospital controls, but could not be replicated with community controls. Odds ratios for allergies tend to be small and cluster around 1.0 as would be expected if there were no true association.

8.6 MEDICAL PROCEDURES

8.6.1 Operations

If an infectious agent plays a role in Alzheimer's disease, then various medical procedures might provide an opportunity for infection. However, case-control studies have failed to find associations between Alzheimer's disease and past surgical interventions (Heyman *et al.*, 1985; Amaducci *et al.*, 1986; Chandra *et al.*, 1987a; Broe *et al.*, 1990), blood transfusions (Heyman *et al.*, 1984; Amaducci *et al.*, 1986; Broe *et al.*, 1990) or grafts (Bharucha *et al.*, 1983). Reported odds ratios for these procedures have been consistently small, ranging from 0.24 to 1.25, arguing strongly against any association.

8.6.2 General anaesthetics

General anaesthetics could plausibly compromise brain function and so predispose to Alzheimer's disease. However, negative results have been reported in four case-control studies (Heyman *et al.*, 1984; Amaducci *et al.*, 1986; Graves *et al.*, 1987; Broe *et al.*, 1990) and odds ratios have been close to 1.0.

8.7 MEDICATION USE

8.7.1 Analgesics

Murray *et al.* (1971) reported neuropathological observations on the brains of nine individuals who had been abusers of analgesics. Seven of these had abused analgesics containing phenacetin, while two had abused aspirin. No pathological changes were observed in the aspirin abusers, but six of the phenacetin abusers had senile plaques and four had neurofibrillary tangles. Since all but one of the phenacetin abusers were aged under 65 at the time of death, these changes were unlikely to be coincidental. Murray *et al.* (1971) argued that these neuropathological changes were due to the effects of phenacetin rather than to renal failure, because similar changes were not seen in patients with chronic renal failure not due to phenacetin abuse. In a separate study of cognitive function in eight analgesic abusers, Murray *et al.* (1971) found definite dementia in four (aged 48–60 years) and possible dementia in a further two.

While Murray *et al.*'s (1971) study provides some evidence of a link between phenacetin abuse and Alzheimer's disease, case-control studies have failed to confirm this association. Heyman *et al.* (1984) found an odds ratio of 1.23 for analgesic use, Broe *et al.* (1990) found an odds ratio of only 0.73, and Amaducci *et al.* (1986) found odds ratios of 1.21 and 1.00 comparing cases to hospital and community controls respectively. It may be that Alzheimer's disease only results in extreme cases of analgesic abuse and these may not have been represented in the case-control studies. A cohort study of analgesic abusers is needed to evaluate properly this potential risk factor.

8.7.2 Antacids

Antacids are of interest as a potential risk factor because many of them contain aluminium. They could thus be a source of the aluminium found in the cores of senile plaques. Three case-control studies have reported on antacid use. Heyman *et al.* (1984) found an odds ratio of only 0.59 for use of antacids containing aluminium, while Broe *et al.* found an odds ratio of 0.93. Similarly, Amaducci *et al.* (1986) found odds ratios of only 0.50 and 0.00 using hospital and community controls respectively. These studies show that, if anything, cases are less likely to have used antacids than controls.

8.7.3 Antiperspirants

Antiperspirants often contain aluminium and are therefore a possible source of exposure to this metal. Only one case-control study has looked at use of aluminium-containing antiperspirants (Graves *et al.*, 1987) and this found a statistically significant association (odds ratio = 2.1). This association therefore merits further study.

8.8 PERSONAL HABITS

8.8.1 Smoking

Case-control studies looking at smoking are summarized in Table 8.14. It can be seen that only one of the 13 studies yielded statistically

Table 8.14   Summary of case-control studies evaluating smoking as a risk factor

Authors	Year	Odds ratio	Statistical significance
Soininen and Heinonen	1982	< 1.00	No
Pinessi *et al.*	1983	?	No
Heyman *et al.*	1984	≈ 1.00*	No
French *et al.*	1985	?	No
Amaducci *et al.*	1986	1.80† (vs. hospital controls)	No
		1.83† (vs. community controls)	No
Chandra *et al.*	1987a	0.57	No
Ferini-Strambi *et al.*	1987	< 1.00‡	Yes
Graves *et al.*	1987	?	No
Jones *et al.*	1987	1.58	No
Shalat *et al.*	1987	2.00	No
Dewey *et al.*§	1988	0.77	No
Katzman *et al.*	1989	0.37	No
Broe *et al.*	1990	0.64‖	No

* Odds ratio for 1+ pack/day since age 40.
† Odds ratio for 10+ cigarettes/day.
‡ Odds ratio for 'heavy smoking'.
§ Looked at dementia syndrome, rather than Alzheimer's disease specifically.
‖ Odds ratio for 1+ pack/day at some time.

significant results and this found smoking to be *less* common in cases than controls. Balanced against this is a claim of a positive association made in Shalat *et al.*'s (1987) case-control study. In their study, a comparison of smokers versus non-smokers provided a non-significant odds ratio of 2.0 (see Table 8.14). However, breaking down smokers by degree of consumption did produce some association. A significant trend for increased risk of Alzheimer's disease with increased cigarette consumption was observed when the effects of educational level and alcohol consumption were partialled out. However, given that the results of the two positive studies are in opposing directions and that ten studies are negative, it seems unlikely there is a true association. This conclusion is confirmed by Mortimer's (1989) meta-analysis of data on smoking from seven case-control studies. He found a pooled odds ratio of only 1.08 for this exposure.

8.8.2 Alcohol consumption

Alcohol is an intuitively plausible risk factor in that it is a widely abused drug having well-known effects on neural functioning. However, it is extremely difficult to evaluate as a risk factor because the clinical diagnosis of Alzheimer's disease often involves the exclusion of cases who have been alcoholic. Such an exclusion procedure was used in the case-control studies by Heyman *et al.* (1984), French *et al.* (1985), Amaducci *et al.* (1986), Shalat *et al.* (1987) and Broe *et al.* (1990). It is therefore not surprising that these studies have found no association between Alzheimer's disease and alcohol consumption. Other case-control studies have not explicitly mentioned alcoholism as an exclusion criterion, but may have used it anyway. These studies also generally failed to find an association (Soininen and Heinonen, 1982; Pinessi *et al.*, 1983; Barclay *et al.*, 1985c; Graves *et al.*, 1987). The one exception is the study by Ferini-Strambi *et al.* (1987) which found long-lasting drinking of more than 50 g of alcohol per day to be significantly *less* common in cases than controls. An artefact of exclusion criteria may have been responsible for this effect.

8.8.3 Physical inactivity

A physically inactive lifestyle has been investigated as a risk factor in only one case-control study, but produced a statistically significant result. Broe *et al.* (1990) found that cases were more likely to have had a physically inactive lifestyle, both in the ten years preceding the study and earlier in life. Physical inactivity in the immediately preceding ten years is likely to be a prodromal feature of Alzheimer's disease, but earlier physical inactivity cannot be explained so simply. The difference could, however, be due to a recall bias in informants who are perhaps influenced by the cases' current inactivity. Replication of this finding is needed before it is taken too seriously.

8.9.1 Malnutrition

Abalan (1984) has proposed that Alzheimer's disease is due to malnutrition, either through inadequate diet or malabsorption of what is available. For early-onset cases with a family history, he proposed that a genetically-mediated malabsorption is the probable cause. In support of this hypothesis, Abalan (1984) has cited evidence that Alzheimer patients have various nutritional deficiencies, but he also admitted that these could be a consequence of the disease rather than a cause.

Other evidence that malnutrition could be a risk factor comes from studies of individuals who have suffered a prolonged period of starvation, with a normal diet subsequently, and have afterwards developed a dementia. Abalan *et al.* (1985) have reported two such cases which fitted criteria for clinical diagnosis of Alzheimer's disease, but no neuropathological evidence was available. Studies of former prisoners-of-war and concentration camp survivors also provide relevant evidence. Gibberd and Simmonds (1980) reported data on over 4000 former prisoners-of-war who had attended a special clinic for check-ups. Some of these were found to develop neurological disorders many years after their release. In 23 cases, this was described as 'cerebral atrophy with dementia'. Gibberd and Simmonds (1980) speculated that there was a possible relationship between nutritional deprivation and the later development of dementia. However, the incidence of dementia was very low in this series and no control group was studied to see if equivalent cases occasionally arise in the general population. A similar study, involving former concentration camp inmates from Norway, has been reported by Løchen (1968). He did cognitive testing of 193 former inmates referred to a hospital because of vocational or social difficulties. These were compared to a control group with known cerebral atrophy. The cognitive test profile of the two groups was found to be very similar. Løchen concluded that 180 of the 193 former inmates showed intellectual impairment, ranging from slight to severe. However, they were a highly selected group of former concentration camp inmates and over half the cases had suffered head trauma in addition to severe malnutrition.

Somewhat more convincing evidence comes from Thygesen *et al.*'s (1970) study of Danish concentration camp survivors over 20 years after their release. They examined a group of survivors who had been assessed for compensation, as well as a group who had not applied for compensation. Psychological testing indicated intellectual deterioration in 61% of the former group and 23% of the latter. As well, 49% of the compensation applicants were clinically evaluated as demented. Intellectual deterioration was found to be more likely in those who were older at the time of imprisonment, those who had suffered greater weight loss, and those from unskilled occupations. The high rate of intellectual impairment in these cases and the association with weight loss argue for malnutrition as the cause. However, other explanations are possible, because concentration camp victims suffered far more than malnutrition. Thygesen *et al.* (1970) reported that head trauma was common and this could account for some or all of the intellectual deterioration. Another possibility is that torture itself has a direct role. Jensen *et al.* (1982) reported that definite cerebral atrophy was found on the CT scans of a number of young and previously healthy torture victims. In only one of their cases was starvation part of the torture.

Even accepting that some aspect of the concentration camp experience produces intellectual deterioration, there is presently no evidence that Alzheimer neuropathology underlies this deterioration. It could be that there is a malnutrition-related dementia which is separate from Alzheimer's disease. Only neuropathological studies will settle this issue.

Only one case-control study of Alzheimer's disease has examined malnutrition as a risk factor. Broe *et al.* (1990) found a non-significant odds ratio of 1.46 for this exposure. However, further case-control studies are needed before any definitive conclusions are drawn about malnutrition.

8.9.2 Dietary sources of infection

If an infectious agent plays a role in Alzheimer's disease, it could enter the body through the eating of infected animals. Accordingly, a number of case-control studies have enquired about possible dietary sources of infection. No associations have been found with eating raw meat (Heyman *et al.*, 1984; French *et al.*, 1985; Chandra *et al.*, 1987a), eating animal brains (Heyman *et al.*, 1984; French *et al.*, 1985) or eating raw seafood (Heyman *et al.*, 1984). Odds ratios for these exposures, where reported, have been low.

8.9.3 Tea and coffee

Coriat and Gillard (1986) have claimed that tea leaves have a high aluminium content and that tea drinking is a major source of aluminium in the British diet. They recommended that tea drinking be avoided by those suffering from Alzheimer's disease and other disorders related to high aluminium levels. However, Fairweather-Tait *et al.* (1987) were unable to replicate these results, finding only a tenth of the aluminium concentration reported by Coriat and Gillard (1986). Furthermore, they argued that the bioavailability of aluminium is an important issue, because the extent to which aluminium is absorbed from the intestinal tract may depend on its chemical form.

Tea, like coffee, is also a source of caffeine which, being a psychoactive drug, could plausibly have some long-term effect on the nervous system. However, case-control studies on both tea and coffee consumption have failed to find an association with Alzheimer's disease (Heyman *et al.*, 1984; French *et al.*, 1985; Broe *et al.*, 1990).

8.9.4 Aluminium cooking utensils

Levick (1980) has proposed that corrosion of aluminium cooking pots could provide a dietary source of aluminium and thus increase the risk for Alzheimer's disease. However, Trapp and Cannon (1981) and Koning (1981) have found that aluminium pots are not an important source of aluminium in the diet. Cooking of acidic foods increase the corrosion of aluminium cookware, but even this effect is not of dietary significance.

Tennakone and Wickramanayake (1987a) have reported that the presence of fluoride in water used for cooking enhances the concentration of aluminium in food a thousand fold. However, this effect could not be replicated by Savory *et al.* (1987) who found only minimal enhancement. Later, Tennakone and Wickramanayake (1987b) themselves reported that they could not reproduce their earlier results.

Aluminium coffee pots have been studied as a particular source of dietary aluminium by Lione *et al.* (1984) and Jackson *et al.* (1989). Both studies found that the pots added a significant amount of aluminium to the beverage. However, as noted above, coffee consumption has not emerged as a risk factor in case-control studies.

Case-control studies have not looked at exposure to aluminium cookware as a potential risk factor, but in view of the small contribution which cookware makes to dietary intake of aluminium, there is little reason to expect an association.

8.9.5 Aluminium in drinking water

Aluminium is largely insoluble in water unless it is acidic. Acid rain in Europe has led to an increase in the aluminium content of drinking water, giving rise to concern that this could affect the incidence of Alzheimer's disease (Pearce, 1985). Evidence for such a link comes from two studies of regional differences in Norway which found that dementia mortality, as assessed from death certificates, was correlated with the aluminium content of the water supply (Vogt, 1986; Flaten, 1987).

However, the validity of using death certificate data to assess dementia mortality has been disputed by Martyn and Pippard (1988) and Jorm *et al.* (1990). Martyn and Pippard (1988) found that only a minority of people diagnosed as demented during life had the diagnosis recorded on their death certificates. Furthermore, regional differences in dementia mortality are influenced by the presence of long-stay institutions in certain regions. Jorm *et al.* (1990) found that death certification practices of particular medical practitioners could have a marked impact on regional differences.

A different approach to the role of aluminium in drinking water has been taken by Martyn *et al.* (1989) in Britain. They assessed the incidence of Alzheimer's disease in 88 districts of England and Wales using records from CT scan units. The study was confined to cases aged under 70 on the assumption that such cases would be highly likely to receive a CT scan. Districts where the concentration of aluminium in water exceeded 0.11 mg/l were found to have a 50% higher incidence than districts where the concentration was only 0–0.01 mg/l. However, there was no clear dose–response relationship. Furthermore, the validity of CT scan records as indicators of regional incidence remains unknown and there has been some questioning of this methodology (Ebrahim, 1989; Lindesay, 1989; Taylor and Davakumar, 1989). Another difficulty is that, even in districts with the highest exposure, drinking water would contribute only a small percentage of total dietary intake. Martyn *et al.*'s (1989) explanation is that the bioavailability of aluminium from drinking water may be greater than from other sources, but this remains to be tested.

A different approach to the issue was taken by Wood *et al.* (1988). They hypothesized that Alzheimer's disease could be related to both

Table 8.15 Summary of the current state of knowledge about risk factors for Alzheimer's disease

Status	Factor	Notes
Confirmed risk factors	Old age	
	Family history of dementia	More important for early-onset Alzheimer's disease
	Down's syndrome	Risk factor for Alzheimer neuropathology only
Possible risk factors	Many ulnar loops	May be more important for early-onset Alzheimer's disease or for males
	Head trauma	
	Family history of Down's syndrome	The size of the effect may be weak

Table 8.15 *continued*

Status	Factor	Notes
Needing further investigation	Sex	
	Race and nationality	
	Family history of haematological malignancies	
	Handedness	
	Advanced maternal age	
	Advanced paternal age	
	Reduced fertility	
	Solvent exposure	
	Use of vibratory tools	
	Encephalitis and meningitis	
	Heart disease	
	Kidney disease	
	Sleep apnoea	
	Phenacetin abuse	
	Alcohol consumption	
	Physical inactivity	
	Malnutrition	
	Aluminium in drinking water	
	Antiperspirant use	
Unlikely risk factors	Birth order	
	Animal exposures	
	Travel in South Pacific	
	Thyroid disease	
	Diabetes	
	Herpes infection	
	Stomach ulcers	
	Arthritis	
	Allergies	
	Operations	
	General anaesthetics	
	Antacid use	
	Smoking	
	Tea and coffee consumption	
	Aluminium cooking utensils	
	Eating raw meat or animal brains	

increased aluminium intake and a negative calcium balance. One group with a negative calcium balance is elderly people suffering from osteoporosis. Accordingly, Wood *et al.* studied elderly patients with hip fractures from two areas with very different aluminium concentrations in the water supply. They found a similar incidence of hip fracture in the two areas and no difference in mental test scores between patients from these areas. These results do not support the hypothesis that aluminium in drinking water is a risk factor for dementia.

Epidemiological field studies of incidence or prevalence are needed to determine properly whether regional differences exist and whether these are correlated with aluminium in drinking water. Such studies presently do not exist, so no conclusion can be reached on aluminium in the water supply as a possible risk factor for Alzheimer's disease.

8.10 SUMMARY OF RISK FACTORS FOR ALZHEIMER'S DISEASE

The foregoing review of evidence on risk factors reveals a complex picture. Nevertheless, some will want a simple answer to the question 'What are the risk factors for Alzheimer's disease?' Table 8.15 attempts to provide a simple answer by listing potential risk factors according to the level of certainty of the presently available evidence. 'Certainty' is very much a subjective assessment and another reviewer might well come up with a different classification.

At this stage, only three risk factors can be regarded as confirmed: old age, family history of dementia and Down's syndrome. The last is a risk factor for Alzheimer neuropathology, but not necessarily for Alzheimer dementia. The 'possible' risk factors have some evidence supporting them, but further investigation is needed to confirm them as risk factors. Some potential risk factors have been classed as 'needing further investigation' either because the existing evidence is mixed (e.g. family history of haematological malignancies), too little work has been done on the topic (e.g. use of vibratory tools), or methodological problems have precluded proper investigation so far (e.g. alcohol consumption). Lastly, there is a group of factors which have been reasonably well researched, but have turned out consistently negative. These can be regarded as not being risk factors at all, or having such a small association with Alzheimer's disease as to be of no practical significance.

9 Theories of Alzheimer's disease: epidemiological contributions

Although the aetiology of Alzheimer's disease is not understood, several plausible theories have been proposed. The development of these theories has been more influenced by advances in the basic biomedical sciences and by clinical observations than by epidemiological findings. Nevertheless, the epidemiological evidence has considerable implications for the viability of these theories. A useful theory of Alzheimer's disease should be able to account for the 'confirmed' risk factors reviewed in the previous chapter, and perhaps also be consistent with some of the 'possible' risk factors. It should not predict positive associations with any of the 'unlikely' risk factors. The purpose of this chapter is to review how well current theories account for this epidemiological evidence.

Five classes of theory are reviewed: **genetic, toxic exposure, infectious agent, free radical**, and **ageing–environment interaction** theories of Alzheimer's disease. In some cases, these classes incorporate several different theories which nevertheless have broad similarities.

9.1 GENETIC THEORIES

9.1.1 Possible genetic mechanisms

There seems little doubt that genetic factors are important in Alzheimer's disease. In recent years, there have been important advances in molecular biological research on genetic factors in Alzheimer's disease. These advances have been in two main areas: the genetic basis of amyloid formation, and single gene effects in familial Alzheimer's disease.

The amyloid found in the cores of senile plaques is known to contain a protein, variously called β or A4, which derives from a larger precursor. The gene for this precursor has been located on chromosome 21 (Goldgaber *et al.*, 1987; Robakis *et al.*, 1987; Tanzi *et al.*, 1987a). The presence of amyloid in the brains of Down's individuals at an early age has been ascribed to the presence of an extra copy of this gene (St George-Hyslop *et al.*, 1987a). There was even the suggestion that three copies of this gene were found in Alzheimer's disease through duplication of a segment of chromosome 21 (Delabar *et al.*, 1987), but later work could not confirm this claim (Podlisny *et al.*, 1987; St George-Hyslop *et al.*, 1987a).

A gene on chromosome 21 has also been implicated in some families which have apparent autosomal dominant transmission of Alzheimer's disease (St George-Hyslop *et al.*, 1987b; Goate *et al.*, 1989). Although it initially seemed possible that this familial gene and the amyloid precursor gene were one and the same, this turned out not to be the case (Tanzi *et al.*, 1987b; Van Broeckhoven *et al.*, 1987). Location of both the amyloid-precursor gene and a familial Alzheimer's disease gene on chromosome 21 appears to be coincidental. How this familial gene works is unknown, but it could be an abnormal promoter of the amyloid-precursor gene. More recently, it has been shown that other cases of familial Alzheimer's disease do not involve linkage to chromosome 21. These cases have been both early-onset (Schellenburg *et al.*, 1988) and late-onset (Roses *et al.*, 1989). It is therefore possible that more than one gene can give rise to familial Alzheimer's disease. In fact, Roses *et al.* (1989) have argued that the Alzheimer's disease gene on chromosome 21 may only be involved in one rare form of the disease. There is presently no evidence that it has a role in the majority of cases, which are of late-onset.

As well as these advances from molecular biology, there has been parallel work using the more traditional genetic method of studying family history of disease. Much of this work has led to the hypothesis of autosomal dominant inheritance. This mode of inheritance was first suggested in the classic study of senile dementia by Larsson *et al.* (1963) and has undergone a revival in recent times. Most of the work supporting autosomal dominant inheritance has relied on estimates of lifetime risk, i.e. the cumulative incidence of Alzheimer's disease up to some age limit (see Chapter 5 for a discussion of the concept of lifetime risk). If Alzheimer's disease is inherited in an autosomal dominant manner, then the lifetime risk to first-degree relatives should be slightly above 50%. The degree to which it is above 50% depends on the frequency of disease-related genes in the population. Breitner and Folstein (1984) and Breitner *et al.* (1986) have proposed that most cases of Alzheimer's disease are due to autosomal dominant inheritance and that these are distinguished from other Alzheimer's disease cases by the presence of language disorder. The lifetime risk in first-degree relatives of cases with language disorder was found to be over 50% by age 90. These results are shown in Figure 9.1.

Similar findings have emerged in other studies, even when there has been no selection for the presence of language disorder (Huff *et al.*, 1988; Martin *et al.*, 1988; Mohs *et al.*, 1987; Zubenko *et al.*, 1988). Such findings have been interpreted as supporting autosomal dominant inheritance for all cases of Alzheimer's disease. However, the findings of all these

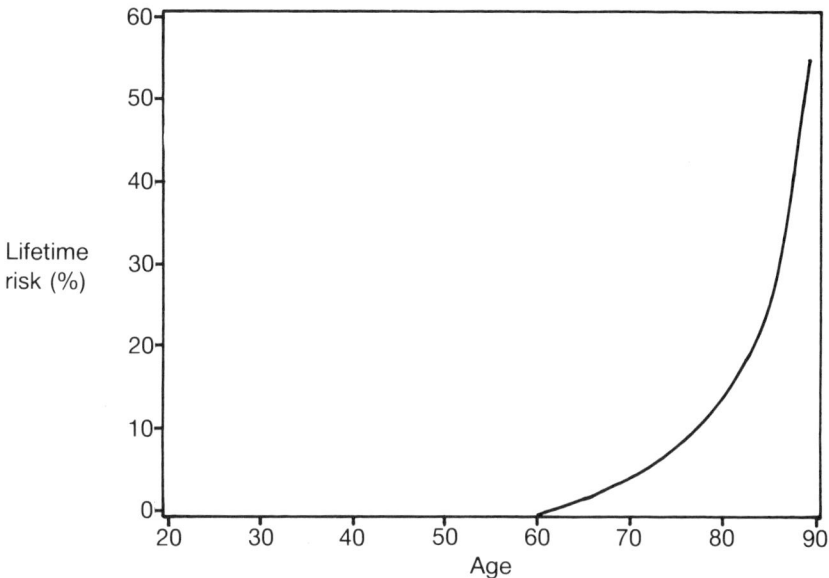

Figure 9.1   Lifetime risk for Alzheimer's disease in first-degree relatives of cases with language disorders. Adapted from Breitner and Folstein (1984).

studies are, in fact, ambiguous. The autosomal dominant hypothesis predicts that lifetime risk for Alzheimer's disease in first-degree relatives will asymptote at slightly over 50%. In other words, once the high risk period of life is past, all carriers should be affected and there should be no incident cases in the remaining relatives. The lifetime risk studies to date, however, show no trend towards an asymptote. Unfortunately, since so few relatives live past age 90, it is extremely difficult to estimate risk beyond this age. If the rising lifetime risk curves to age 90 are projected to older ages, the risk would be substantially more than 50%. In fact, the available data are equally compatible with the hypothesis that *all* first-degree relatives will be affected if they live long enough. This possibility is clearly evident in Figure 9.1, where the cumulative incidence rises in an exponential manner and might feasibly reach 100% at some extreme old age. Contrast this with Figure 9.2 which shows the lifetime risk to first-degree relatives of Huntington's disease cases. Huntington's disease is a well-known autosomal disorder and shows a clear asymptote at 50% risk for first-degree relatives.

Further support for autosomal dominant inheritance comes from work by Zubenko *et al.* (1987) in which they studied platelet membrane fluidity in Alzheimer's disease cases and their relatives. They found

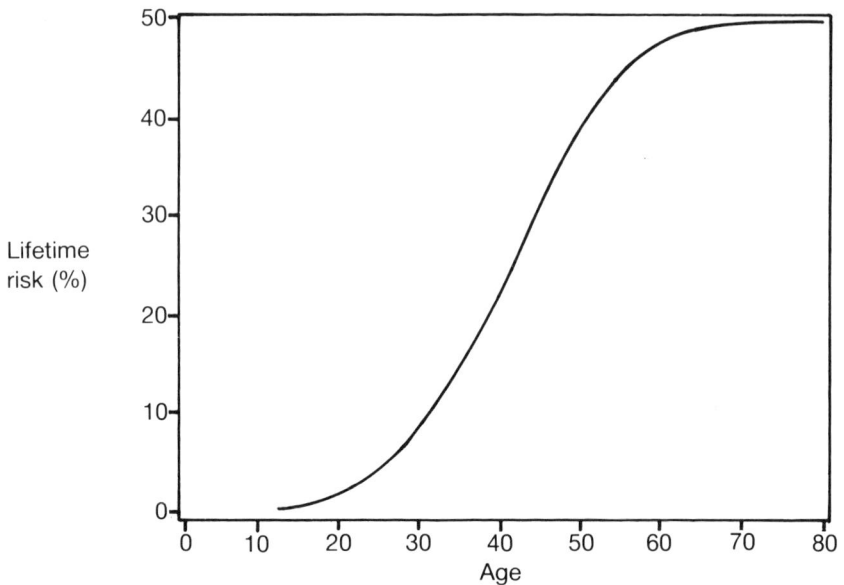

Figure 9.2 Lifetime risk for Huntington's disease in first-degree relatives of cases. Based on data from Heston and White (1983).

platelet membrane fluidity to be abnormal in a subgroup of Alzheimer's disease patients and also in around 50% of first-degree relatives who were not yet affected by Alzheimer's disease. On the basis of these findings, Zubenko et al. (1987) hypothesized that abnormal platelet membrane fluidity is a genetic marker for familial Alzheimer's disease and is transmitted in an autosomal dominant manner. Later, Zubenko et al. (1988) studied lifetime risk in first-degree relatives of Alzheimer's disease patients with and without platelet membrane abnormality. They found approximately 50% risk up to age 90 in both groups, with the abnormal membrane fluidity group simply having earlier onset. They hypothesized either a single gene for Alzheimer's disease which has its expression modified by abnormal platelet membrane fluidity or else two Alzheimer's disease genes, one of which is linked to abnormal platelet membrane fluidity.

In contrast to the simple autosomal dominant hypothesis, Wright and Whalley (1984) proposed a more complex mechanism. They argued that there is a rare subgroup of early-onset Alzheimer's disease cases with autosomal dominant inheritance, while late-onset cases appear to be associated with early cerebral ageing. Complex genetic factors influence this rate of ageing. If late-onset Alzheimer's disease is part of the ageing process, then the lifetime risk should asymptote at 100%, rather than the 50% predicted by the single gene hypothesis.

9.1.2 Consistency with epidemiological findings

Genetic theories successfully explain many of the risk factors for Alzheimer's disease. The rapid rise in incidence with age can be seen as the expression of an age-dependent genetic mechanism. In terms of the autosomal dominant hypothesis, incidence would be predicted to rise initially with age, but later fall as carriers of the gene make up a progressively smaller proportion of the survivors. It should not be uncommon for extremely old individuals to be unaffected by Alzheimer's disease. If, by contrast, Alzheimer's disease is an intrinsic part of the ageing process which is labelled as a disease in those cases where it occurs unusually early, people unaffected by Alzheimer's disease should be rare amongst the extremely elderly.

Family history of dementia as a risk factor is readily accommodated by genetic theories. The autosomal dominant hypothesis predicts that Alzheimer's disease should be present in around 50% of first-degree relatives provided they live through the at-risk period. The 'normal ageing' hypothesis also predicts some familial association because there are many genes thought to have an influence on the rate of ageing (Wright and Whalley, 1984).

The various links with Down's syndrome are likewise readily amenable to a genetic interpretation. The presence of Alzheimer neuropathology from middle-age on in Down's syndrome suggests that genes on chromosome 21 play an important role. Indeed, with the localization of the amyloid-precursor gene on this chromosome, a simple gene-dosage effect appears a plausible explanation. However, given the dissociation between neuropathology and dementia in Down's syndrome, genes on chromosome 21 may be sufficient for the production of plaques and tangles but not for major cognitive decline.

The other Alzheimer's disease risk factors suggesting an association with Down's – ulnar loops and family history of Down's syndrome – could also be explained by genetic factors, but the potential mechanisms are unclear. One possibility is that some early-onset cases of Alzheimer's disease are, in fact, undetected Down's mosaics (Rowe *et al.*, 1989). This would explain the presence of Alzheimer neuropathology at an early age, the frequency of ulnar loops and Down's syndrome in relatives. There is, however, no direct evidence for this hypothesis.

While genetic effects are clearly important in Alzheimer's disease, they cannot provide a complete account. Cases of monozygotic twins discordant for Alzheimer's disease (Nee *et al.*, 1987; Creasey *et al.*, 1989) show that environmental factors also play a role. While there are as yet no established environmental risk factors for Alzheimer's disease, head trauma is a possible one.

9.2 TOXIC EXPOSURE THEORIES

9.2.1 The aluminium theory

The toxic substance which has received pre-eminent attention as a possible cause of Alzheimer's disease is aluminium. There are important pieces of evidence suggesting a possible role for aluminium in Alzheimer's disease. Aluminosilicates are present in the cores of senile plaques, with aluminium comprising 4–19% of the centre of the core (Edwardson *et al.*, 1986). Furthermore, aluminium has been found to accumulate in neurones containing neurofibrillary tangles. While aluminium clearly has an important role, there is considerable dispute about whether it is a cause of plaque and tangle formation or a secondary accumulation.

The traditional view of plaque formation is that they go through several stages, beginning with swollen neurites lacking a plaque core and ending with only the core remaining (Terry and Wisniewski, 1970). This theory relegates aluminium to a secondary role because it is present in the plaque cores. By contrast, others have argued that amyloid and its associated aluminosilicates initiate the formation of plaques, even though early plaques may lack an obvious core (Edwardson *et al.*, 1986).

Animal studies have been carried out to establish a causal role for aluminium in tangle formation. Klatzo *et al.* (1965) found that direct application of aluminium salts to the brain could produce a type of neurofibrillary degeneration in rabbits and cats. However, the structure of these neurofilaments is different to that seen in Alzheimer's disease. A possible explanation is that Alzheimer neurofibrillary tangles do not occur naturally in these species. Aluminium might still produce Alzheimer changes in the human brain. However, Foncin (1987) has reported a case of accidental metallic aluminium implantation in the human brain. While this implantation produced toxic effects, Alzheimer neuropathology did not result. Similarly, McLaughlin *et al.* (1962) reported on a worker who developed a rapidly progressive encephalopathy after working in an aluminium powder factory for 13.5 years. Although his brain was found to contain 17 times the normal amount of aluminium, there was no Alzheimer neuropathology at post-mortem. Further relevant evidence comes from cases of dialysis dementia in which high concentrations of aluminium are found in the brain (McDermott and Smith, 1978). Dialysis patients are exposed to increased levels of aluminium because of the large quantity of water used in dialysis and the use of phosphate-binding gels which contain aluminium. However, dialysis dementia is neuropathologically distinct from Alzheimer's disease and presents a different clinical picture (Greenhouse, 1982).

If aluminium were to play a role in the aetiology of Alzheimer's disease, it must enter the brain in some way. The most obvious possibility is through the diet, but the bioavailability of aluminium in the diet is believed to be low. Using rats, Mayor *et al.* (1977) have found that the gastrointestinal absorption of aluminium and its deposition in the brain is greatly increased by parathyroid hormone. This finding suggested that Alzheimer's disease might result from parathyroid hormone acting on orally ingested aluminium. However, Shore and Wyatt (1983) were unable to find any difference between Alzheimer's disease patients and controls in parathyroid hormone or in aluminium concentration in serum, cerebrospinal fluid or hair. An obstacle to the deposition of aluminium in the brain is, of course, the blood–brain barrier. Edwardson *et al.* (1986) have proposed that Alzheimer's disease involves a lesion, which may be genetic or environmental in origin, predisposing affected individuals to breakdown of the blood–brain barrier for aluminium. Once this breakdown has occurred, deposition in the brain would also be affected by the degree of environmental exposure to aluminium.

Another possible source of entry, besides the gastrointestinal tract, is along nasal-olfactory pathways. Roberts (1986) and Perl and Good (1987) have proposed that Alzheimer's disease involves a defect of the olfactory mucosa or olfactory bulb barriers, leading to the entry of aluminium-containing compounds to the brain. Perl and Good (1987) have supported this proposal by an experiment on rabbits in which aluminium salts were deposited in the nasal recesses. This exposure produced granulomatous lesions, but did not result in the type of neurofibrillary changes seen after intracerebral exposure to aluminium. Other evidence for the possible importance of nasal-olfactory pathways in Alzheimer's disease comes from neuropathological studies showing neurofibrillary tangles to be present in the olfactory bulbs (Esiri and Wilcock, 1984) and abnormalities in the sensory epithelium of the nose (Talamo *et al.*, 1989). The olfactory sense is also impaired early in Alzheimer's disease, but this seems to be a problem of olfactory recognition rather than olfactory detection (Koss *et al.*, 1988), suggesting that the primary impairment is central rather than peripheral. Exactly how aluminium could naturally find its way up the olfactory pathway to the brain has not been fully specified. Roberts (1986) has claimed that aluminosilicates are very common in the environment and can be breathed in as dust. However, the exposure of the olfactory system through inhalation must be very small in normal circumstances.

9.2.2 Consistency with epidemiological findings

The aluminium-exposure theory could explain old age as a risk factor in terms of the elderly having had greater duration of exposure. There might also be age-related breakdown of the barriers to entry of aluminium into the brain – the olfactory mucosa and/or the blood–brain barrier.

Family history of dementia as a risk factor could reflect a genetic predisposition to breakdown of barriers to the entry of aluminium. There is, however, no direct evidence of such a genetic mechanism. Another possibility is that familial clustering occurs because of a shared environmental exposure to aluminium. However, if the adult environment is crucial, then spouses would be expected to have increased risk because of their shared living arrangements, but the evidence does not support this.

The link of Alzheimer neuropathology to Down's syndrome is not readily explained, but there could be some gene on chromosome 21 which, in triplicate, leads to breakdown of barriers to aluminium. Again, while this is a possibility, there is no direct evidence to support it.

The effects of head trauma could be accommodated within an aluminium-exposure theory if it were assumed that the trauma disrupted the blood–brain barrier and allowed aluminium to enter. Other possible risk factors (ulnar loops and family history of Down's) are, however, not readily incorporated within an aluminium theory.

Environmental exposure to aluminium is clearly predicted to be a risk factor under this theory. However, dietary exposure to aluminium-containing antacids is clearly not a risk factor, and use of aluminium cookware is believed to result in a very small increase in exposure. Exposure to aluminium in the water supply, particularly where this is enhanced through acid rain, has been proposed as a risk factor, but the evidence on which this is based is of doubtful validity. One case-control study (Graves *et al.*, 1987) has implicated exposure to aluminium-containing antiperspirants, but this finding needs replication before being taken too seriously. Interestingly, hypotheses that aluminium toxicity is a factor in Alzheimer's disease have not considered absorption through the skin as a possible mechanism of exposure. Olfactory exposure to aluminium, which has been proposed as a possible mechanism, has not been considered in risk factor studies, but it is unclear exactly how such an exposure could be ascertained.

All in all, the aluminium theory finds only weak support in either the experimental or epidemiological evidence. The only solid ground on which the theory rests is the observed concentration of aluminium in the core of senile plaques and in neurofibrillary tangle-bearing neurones. To accommodate other evidence of an apparently contradictory nature, various unsatisfying post-hoc explanations have to be put forward.

9.2.3 Other toxic exposures

While there is little support for the theory that aluminium exposure causes Alzheimer's disease, other toxic exposures are possible. The only other toxic exposure for which some supporting evidence exists is phenacetin. This evidence comes from Murray *et al.*'s (1971) observation of Alzheimer neuropathology and intellectual deterioration in phenacetin abusers. However, other studies looking at analgesic use have failed to find evidence of this as a risk factor, although these studies may not have included extreme abusers of the sort examined by Murray *et al.* (1971). Given that phenacetin abuse is a fairly rare occurrence, it could at best be only a minor cause of Alzheimer's disease and could not possibly account for all the existing epidemiological knowledge of the disease. However, if phenacetin abuse did turn out to produce Alzheimer's disease, then an understanding of the mechanisms involved could lead to the discovery of other environmental exposures which have similar effects. Murray *et al.* (1971) suggested that phenacetin produced accelerated brain ageing by overwhelming the body's antioxidant protection. This possibility is considered later in this chapter when discussing the free radical theory.

9.3 INFECTIOUS AGENT THEORIES

9.3.1 The unconventional virus theory

The idea that Alzheimer's disease is due to an infectious agent would seem unlikely if it were not for the discovery that certain other neurological diseases are transmissible. There are three known transmissible neurological disorders in humans: kuru, Creutzfeldt–Jakob disease and Gerstmann–Sträussler syndrome.

Transmission was first demonstrated with kuru, a rare degenerative neurological disease found in a region of Papua New Guinea (Gajdusek, 1977). The disease has been successfully transmitted to chimpanzees and other primates. In humans, transmission of the disease was associated with the ritual cannibalism of dead kinsman which was practised in certain regions of Papua New Guinea. This practice often resulted in brain tissue being smeared on bodies. The incidence of the disease has declined dramatically as this traditional practice has been abandoned.

The transmissibility of Creutzfeldt–Jakob disease was demonstrated soon after that of kuru. It is a rare dementing disorder with a worldwide distribution. In some cases it appears to be familial and in others sporadic. Instances of human transmission have been documented as occurring through transplant of affected tissue and use of infected medical instruments (Gajdusek, 1977). Gerstmann–Sträussler syndrome is a rare chronic cerebellar ataxia which may be a variant of Creutzfeldt–Jakob disease (Masters *et al.*, 1981). It has also been transmitted to animals.

A disease related to Creutzfeldt–Jakob disease, but not known to affect humans, is scrapie. It occurs naturally in sheep and goats and has been transmitted to other species such as mice and hamsters. When goats are infected with Creutzfeldt–Jakob disease from humans, the resulting disease is indistinguishable from natural scrapie (Prusiner, 1982).

The above diseases are due to previously unknown infectious agents which Gajdusek (1977) has called 'unconventional viruses'. These have properties different in many ways from conventional viruses. Amongst their unusual properties are a long incubation period (up to decades), none of the inflammatory responses usually associated with viral infections, and resistance to deactivation by physical and chemical means effective for conventional viruses. Prusiner (1982) has hypothesized that these infectious agents consist of a protein devoid of nucleic acid, and dubbed them 'prions' (short for proteinaceous infectious agents). If prions lack a nucleic acid, then previously unknown methods of replication must be involved. The prion hypothesis remains controversial.

While the transmissible neurological diseases might be seen as having an environmental origin, Ridley *et al.* (1986) have concluded that this is not so in the majority of cases. They argued that, in most cases, these diseases arise from a sequence in the genome and are genetically transmitted. The distinction between genetic and infectious aetiologies is blurred by their proposal that certain genes may be expressed as infectious particles. Ridley *et al.* (1986) hypothesized that such genes are expressed as infectious particles by some unspecified age-dependent process and give rise to 'sporadic' cases. In some families there is a genetic predisposition to such an age-dependent expression and familial cases of the disease are the result. In the extreme, the genetic risk of expression can give rise to an autosomal dominant pattern of familial disease.

Given the similarities of the infectious neurological diseases to Alzheimer's disease, there has been speculation that it too could be due to an unconventional virus. Gajdusek (1977) has conjectured that the scrapie agent may have been the origin for Creutzfeldt–Jakob disease, kuru and familial Alzheimer's disease. The scrapie agent is known to be modified by different hosts so that, for example, when primates are infected by scrapie virus from sheep, goats or mice, the virus cannot be re-infected back to the species from which it originated. Thus, kitchen or butchery accidents could have led to infection of humans which took the form of Creutzfeldt–Jakob disease. A sporadic case of Creutzfeldt–Jakob disease in Papua New Guinea may have given rise to the kuru epidemic through the practice of endocannibalism. Creutzfeldt–Jakob disease might in turn have given rise to familial Alzheimer's disease through some unknown sourse of transmission. Prusiner (1984) has also proposed that Alzheimer's disease is transmissible and has even suggested that amyloid deposits represent accumulations of Alzheimer's disease prions.

The ultimate test of the theory that Alzheimer's disease is due to an unconventional virus is to demonstrate transmissibility. Early attempts to transmit the disease to animals were largely unsuccessful. The only exception was two cases reported by Goudsmit *et al.* (1980) in which inocula made from the brains of patients with familial Alzheimer's disease produced a disease like Creutzfeldt–Jakob disease in monkeys. However, attempts to replicate these results were unsuccessful, even with inoculation from the same two familial cases. These failures do not necessarily rule out a role for an infectious agent. As Prusiner (1984) has pointed out, animals may not be susceptible to the agent or the incubation time could be so long that the disease does not manifest within the lifespan of experimental animals. Recently, positive evidence for transmissibility has come from a study by Manuelidis *et al.* (1988) using a new approach. They hypothesized that Alzheimer's disease might be infective only in its early stages, hence the general failure to demonstrate transmission with post-mortem tissue. Because brain tissue is not available in the early stages of Alzheimer's disease, Manuelidis *et al.* (1988) used the buffy coat of blood, which earlier work had shown could contain the Creutzfeldt–Jakob disease agent. Using the blood of both Alzheimer's disease patients and their as yet unaffected relatives, transmission was produced in a number of hamsters and could be transmitted from these to new hamsters. This transmission produced a spongiform encephalopathy which could not be distinguished from Creutzfeldt–Jakob disease. Manuelidis *et al.* (1988) speculated that Alzheimer's disease and Creutzfeldt–Jakob disease are caused by the same agent, with host factors producing Creutzfeldt–Jakob disease in rare instances, but Alzheimer's disease in most. In animals, only Creutzfeldt–Jakob disease is seen because Alzheimer neuropathology cannot be expressed. While these results and ideas are very exciting, they require replication from others before the transmissibility of Alzheimer's disease can be taken seriously. There is other evidence that Creutzfeldt–Jakob disease and Alzheimer's disease are not linked. Roberts *et al.* (1986) tried to stain amyloid plaques in Creutzfeldt–Jakob disease and Alzheimer's disease with prion-protein antiserum derived from scrapie-infected animals. Staining was successful in cases of Creutzfeldt–Jakob disease, kuru and Gerstmann-Sträussler syndrome, but not in Alzheimer's disease. These results suggest that the scrapie or Creutzfeldt–Jakob agents do not cause Alzheimer's disease.

9.3.2 The conventional virus theory

It is not only unconventional viruses which can give rise to chronic neurological diseases after long incubation periods. Gajdusek (1977) has listed many such diseases caused by conventional viruses. It is therefore possible that Alzheimer's disease is also caused by the reactivation of a conventional virus. The particular virus which has been proposed as a possible cause of Alzheimer's disease is herpes simplex. Ball (1982) has hypothesized that herpes simplex virus can be latent in human trigeminal ganglia. The virus can travel down the neural pathway to produce labial herpes or up to the limbic system to cause acute or chronic brain disease. The acute form is herpes simplex encephalitis, but if there is partial resistance to the virus the result can be Alzheimer's disease. The anatomical links between the trigeminal ganglia and the limbic system are hypothesized to account for the early occurrence of Alzheimer neuropathology in this region. Esiri (1982) has put forward a similar hypothesis. She has proposed that herpes simplex virus produces a latent infection of the olfactory bulbs and associated neural pathways. In most cases, this infection has no immediate consequences, but in old age the metabolism of these neurones is affected and neurofibrillary tangles develop. Where the distribution of these changes is more widespread, Alzheimer's disease is the result. This theory predicts that the pathways of the virus into the brain should be the first affected. Esiri and Wilcock (1984) have observed that the olfactory pathway is affected by neurofibrillary tangles in Alzheimer's disease and Talamo *et al.* (1989) have found abnormalities in the sensory epithelium of the nose. Ulrich (1985) has attempted to ascertain the origin of Alzheimer neuropathology by studying non-demented people dying in late middle age. Three-quarters of his sample had plaques or tangles at death. Neurofibrillary tangles were consistently present in the entorhinal cortex and/or hippocampus, while the olfactory bulb was occasionally involved. This pattern of involvement suggested to Ulrich (1985) that any infectious agent was more likely to invade via the trigeminal ganglion than the olfactory mucosa.

9.3.3 Consistency with epidemiological findings

Infectious agent theories can account for old age as a risk factor in terms of the long incubation periods of unconventional viruses and of some conventional viruses. It may only be the elderly who have lived long enough to manifest a disease latent in much of the population.

Family history of dementia as a risk factor can also be interpreted in infectious terms. One possibility is that an infectious agent is transmitted vertically through the genome and horizontally to family members in close contact. Horizontal transmission is, however, less plausible given that spouses of Alzheimer's cases do not have an increased incidence of dementia. Another possibility, argued by Wisniewski *et al.* (1984), is that Alzheimer's disease requires both an infectious agent and a genetically susceptible host. This hypothesis would also predict familial clustering of the disease.

The occurrence of Alzheimer neuropathology in Down's syndrome has been interpreted in terms of an infectious theory. Wisniewski *et al.* (1985) have pointed out that Down's individuals are particularly susceptible to viral infections. This may be connected with the presence of antiviral genes on chromosome 21. There is, of course, no direct evidence to support this speculation.

The possible risk factors – ulnar loops, head trauma and family history of Down's – are not readily incorporated in an infectious agent theory, although it could be hypothesized that head trauma somehow breaks down the brain's barriers to infections. The herpes simplex theory predicts that Alzheimer's disease cases should have a greater frequency of infection with this virus than controls. However, well-designed case-control and immunological studies have been uniformly negative.

If an unconventional virus were responsible for Alzheimer's disease, then it might be acquired through contact with animals or through medical interventions. However, neither exposure to animals, eating raw meat or animal brains, nor a history of invasive medical procedures appear to have any association with Alzheimer's disease. Even the habit of nose picking, which might provide entry for an infectious agent, has been investigated and produced negative results (Broe *et al.*, 1990). Manuelidis *et al.* (1988) have claimed transmission of Alzheimer's disease to animals via the buffy coat of blood, but blood transfusions do not appear to be a risk factor in humans.

Infectious agent theories seem to provide a poor account of the existing epidemiological evidence. Were it not for the recent demonstration of transmissibility in the study by Manuelidis *et al.* (1988), the possibility of an infectious aetiology might be dismissed altogether. A final verdict must await replication of this work. However, if an unconventional virus were involved, it is unlikely to be *the* cause of Alzheimer's disease. Other factors, particularly genetic ones, must play an important role as well.

9.4 THE FREE RADICAL THEORY

Free radicals are atoms or molecules with one or more unpaired electrons in their outer orbit. They are particularly likely to arise in chemical reactions involving oxygen. When oxygen is reduced to water, free radical intermediaries may be formed. These are the superoxide and hydroxyl radicals. These free radicals react with other molecules and create new free radicals, thus setting off a chain reaction. These reactions have highly destructive effects on biological functions. Free radicals have a particular affinity for polysaturated lipids, which are found in all cells, but can also have destructive effects on DNA, proteins and carbohydrates. The body has natural defences against free radicals, including enzymes like superoxide dismutase and antioxidants like vitamin E.

Harman (1985) has proposed that free radical reactions are the cause of ageing and age-related diseases, including Alzheimer's disease. According to this theory, ageing occurs through the progressive accumulation of irreversible damage caused by free radicals. Free radical reactions are modified by various genetic and environmental factors which may sometimes produce patterns of effects so different from normal ageing that they are labelled as a disease. As evidence for the role of free radicals in Alzheimer's disease, Harman (1985) cited the deposition of lipofuscin in the brain. Lipofuscin is formed by the oxidative degradation of lipids and is a well-known feature of the ageing brain. Harman also gave it an important role in Alzheimer's disease. However, lipofuscin is not generally seen as one of the histopathological hallmarks of Alzheimer's disease. According to Wright and Whalley (1984), some researchers have found increased lipofuscin in the brains of Alzheimer's disease cases, but others have not.

Harman (1985) has also argued that free radicals are involved in the formation of amyloid. In support of this he cited experiments with mice showing that antioxidants inhibited amyloid-formation. Similarly, Beyreuther *et al.* (1988) have speculated that free radicals may play a role in damage to neuronal membranes, allowing the release of the amyloid precursor and its conversion to amyloid.

The role of aluminium in Alzheimer neuropathology has also been interpreted in terms of the action of free radicals by Halliwell and Gutteridge (1986). Iron acts as a catalyst for the production of the hydroxyl radical. While aluminium is unable itself to promote radical reactions, it can accelerate iron-stimulated peroxidation of lipids.

A pathological feature of Alzheimer's disease not readily explained by the free radical theory is increased cell membrane fluidity (Zubenko *et al.*, 1987). Free radicals cause lipid peroxidation which reduces cell membrane fluidity (Halliwell and Gutteridge, 1985), the opposite of what is observed in Alzheimer's disease.

While there is much informed speculation about the potential role of free radicals in Alzheimer's disease, little direct evidence is available. Unfortunately, the presence of free radical reactions in the body is difficult to detect because they are so short-lived. The presence of such reactions is usually inferred from the presence of free-radical scavenging enzymes such as superoxide dismutase. Marklund *et al.* (1985) compared superoxide dismutase in Alzheimer and normal brains and found no difference in any of four brain regions studied, including the hippocampus. In a similar study, Marttila and Rinne (1988) looked at the levels of several antioxidant enzymes in the brains of Alzheimer's disease cases and controls, including superoxide dismutase and glutathione peroxidase. They found a several-fold decrease in superoxide dismutase in the nucleus basalis of Meynert and a slight increase in the substantia nigra, but no differences in frontal or temporal cortex or hippocampus. There was also a slight increase in glutathione perioxidase levels in the nucleus basalis. The failure to find any differences in the hippocampus in either of the above studies is a disturbing inconsistency for the free radical theory since this region is universally affected in Alzheimer's disease. A study of glutathione peroxidase in erythrocytes also showed a significant elevation in Alzheimer's disease, although there was considerable overlap with normals (Anneren *et al.*, 1986). This elevation was interpreted as reflecting an increased production of peroxides within these cells. The relevance of this finding to brain function is, however, unclear.

If Alzheimer's disease sufferers could be clearly shown to differ on free radical scavenging enzymes, the interpretation of the findings would be uncertain. Such a difference might reflect an aetiological role for free radical reactions or could be a secondary effect of neuronal deterioration. Damaged tissue undergoes free radical reactions more readily than healthy tissue and Dormandy (1988) has pointed out the positive role which free radicals have in removing defective cells from the body.

9.4.1 Consistency with epidemiological findings

Henderson (1988) has reviewed the evidence on risk factors for Alzheimer's disease and concluded that the free radical theory can account for much of this evidence, including the increasing risk with age, the association with Down's syndrome, and the effects of head injury and phenacetin abuse. Here we consider the theory's ability to account for the risk factors reviewed in the previous chapter.

The theory accounts for the increased incidence of Alzheimer's disease with age in terms of the progressive accumulation of free-radical induced damage with time. According to Harman (1985), there are likely to be genetic differences between individuals in genes which control free radical reactions and those which defend against free radicals. Such genes might account for family history of dementia as a risk factor for Alzheimer's disease. However, it must be emphasized that Harman (1985) has cited no evidence for such genetic variability, nor is there any evidence that people affected by Alzheimer's disease differ with respect to genes controlling free radicals.

The presence of Alzheimer neuropathology in Down's syndrome has been explained by the presence of the superoxide dismutase gene on chromosome 21. The presence of an extra chromosome in Down's syndrome produces a 50% increase in this enzyme by a gene dosage effect. While the presence of additional superoxide scavenger enzyme might seem advantageous, Sinet (1982) has argued that this enzyme also produces an oxidant, peroxide, which in the presence of iron is converted to the highly destructive hydroxyl radical. It is the hydroxyl radical which is thought to lead to the accelerated ageing effects seen in Down's syndrome, including Alzheimer neuropathology.

Of the 'possible' risk factors, the free radical theory does not account for ulnar loops, but could explain the effect of head injury. According to Halliwell and Gutteridge (1986), injured or diseased tissues undergo free-radical reactions more readily than normal tissues. Thus, free radicals may exacerbate any tissue damage. However, as Dormandy (1988) has argued, this process is not necessarily bad. Free radicals provide an essential service in removing defective cells from the body. The free radical theory does not appear to explain why a period of many years can intervene between an incident of head trauma and the onset of Alzheimer's disease. The action of free radicals should be more immediate.

While the evidence on phenacetin abuse as a risk factor is conflicting, an association is predicted by the free radical theory. Overdose of phenacetin is known to produce lipid peroxidation (Clark *et al.*, 1985) and this could account for the accumulation of lipofuscin in Alzheimer's disease cases associated with phenacetin abuse (Murray *et al.*, 1971).

The free radical theory of Alzheimer's disease is highly speculative. It can account for some of the known facts about the disease, but direct evidence of abnormal free radical activity in Alzheimer's disease is lacking. From an epidemiological perspective, the theory gives a *post hoc* explanation of some important risk factors, but its predictive power needs to be tested. For example, Clark *et al.* (1985) have listed factors which increase free radical activity or decrease the body's protection from free radicals. Such factors need to be examined in epidemiological studies as potential risk factors for Alzheimer's disease.

9.5 THE AGEING AND ENVIRONMENT INTERACTION THEORY

Calne and associates (1986) have proposed that environmental exposures (including trauma, toxins and infectious agents) can cause loss of neurones in specific areas of the central nervous system which do not have clinically significant effects at the time, but compound with the normal loss of neurones which occurs with ageing to produce neurological disorders later in life. There is mounting evidence that a mechanism of this sort operates for a number of neurological diseases, such as Parkinson's disease, the Guam parkinsonism–dementia complex, and post-poliomyelitis syndrome.

With Parkinson's disease, it has been discovered that a toxic chemical, MPTP, can selectively destroy cells in the substantia nigra. Sometimes this destruction produces Parkinson's disease fairly rapidly, but in other cases there may be a delay of many years between exposure to MPTP and onset of the disease. Calne *et al.* (1986) proposed that, in these delayed cases, additional neurones are lost from the substantia nigra with normal ageing so that eventually a critical threshold is reached and symptoms of Parkinson's disease appear. Although exposure to MPTP is probably only a minor cause of Parkinson's disease, it serves as a useful model for how other toxic exposures might work in this disease.

The parkinsonian–dementia complex of Guam is a neurological disease confined to the native people of this island and certain other isolated regions in the Pacific. The disease combines elements of Alzheimer's disease, Parkinson's disease and motoneurone disease. Recently, evidence from animal studies has indicated that the disease could be caused by consumption of the cycad seed (Spencer *et al.*, 1987). This seed appears to contain one or more neurotoxins which may take decades to produce clinically significant effects and have hence been termed 'slow toxins'. There are cases of Guamians who left their homeland for the United States in early adult life and did not thereafter consume cycad seeds. The disease has subsequently appeared after an interval of 30 years.

In the post-poliomyelitis syndrome, motor function may begin to deteriorate many years after infection with the polio virus, and without evidence of subsequent activity by the virus. Again, loss of motor neurones with ageing could be implicated.

In these diseases and others, there is initially some specific loss of neuronal function which may not result in a clinically significant effect. The central nervous system has considerable reserves which allow cells to be lost and their functions to be taken up by other cells. Compensation for loss of neurones can occur through neuronal sprouting, increased rate of neurotransmitter synthesis, and an increased number of receptors. However, as more neurones are lost with ageing, the remainder cannot continue to maintain normal function. Loss of these neurones begins to produce clinically significant effects.

Calne *et al.* (1986) have hypothesized that the aetiology of Alzheimer's disease involves a similar mechanism. According to this hypothesis, the crucial lesion for Alzheimer's disease may be in the cholinergic cells of the basal forebrain. Loss of these cells could then produce secondary effects in other regions of the brain. Basal forebrain cholinergic neurones are known to be lost progressively with ageing. However, dementia would not appear until neuronal reserves and compensatory processes are exhausted. Loss of neurones early in life through trauma, toxic exposures or infection, could hasten the crossing of the threshold for dementia. It is notable that the theory does not specify a single environmental cause for the initial neuronal loss but allows multiple possibilities. Furthermore, the theory does not necessitate that the processes which lead to neuronal death through environmental exposure are the same as those that operate with ageing. In other words, the environmental exposure would not itself have to produce the neuropathological hallmarks of Alzheimer's disease in affected neurones, but could simply magnify the clinical implications of Alzheimer changes occurring in old age.

9.5.1 Consistency with epidemiological findings

The ageing and environment interaction theory does not specify what types of environmental events might predispose people to Alzheimer's disease, simply that such events may occur many decades before onset of the disease. The epidemiological implications are therefore a little vague but point to a search for environmental factors early in life. Of the potential risk factors reviewed in the previous chapter, head trauma is the one which best fits with this theory. Heyman *et al.* (1984) and Mortimer *et al.* (1985a) have reported that the interval between head trauma and onset of Alzheimer's disease is several decades in many cases, with an intervening period in which there are no clinically-significant effects. Given that head trauma may cause loss of neurones from many brain regions, it might be expected to be a risk factor for a range of neurological diseases associated with ageing.

Other risk factors can also be explained in terms of an interaction between ageing and environment. The increasing incidence of Alzheimer's disease with age can be seen as due to the age-associated loss of neurones and the consequently increased probability that neuronal reserves and compensatory mechanisms will be exhausted. Family history of dementia as a risk factor can be interpreted in both environmental and genetic terms. It could reflect common environmental exposures early in life or genetically-mediated individual differences in the susceptibility to these environmental exposures. Other possible risk factors, namely ulnar loops and a family history of Down's, lie essentially outside the scope of the theory.

Obviously, the ageing and environment interaction theory cannot produce a complete account of Alzheimer's disease, but it does not pretend to. The theory has nothing to say about genetically-mediated effects, but tries to account for the possibly delayed action of environmental events.

9.6 CONCLUSION

Although the five theories of Alzheimer's disease discussed in this chapter have been presented as if they are mutually exclusive alternatives, it is readily apparent that they are not. It is also clear that none of these theories can alone provide a full account of the epidemiology of Alzheimer's disease. Several of the theories could be true simultaneously and it is not difficult to sketch an overarching theory incorporating elements of them all. Figure 9.3 shows a general theory which is compatible with the known facts about Alzheimer's disease. This theory allows for both genetic and environmental influences. Genes control ageing of the brain, which is a universal human characteristic. In addition, there are specific genes, carried by only some individuals, which predispose to Alzheimer's disease. These genes give rise to early-onset familial Alzheimer's disease and can show an autosomal dominant pattern of inheritance. A range of environmental factors can also operate, but these are poorly understood at this time. They include unknown toxic exposures, certain infectious agents and trauma to the brain. Both genetic and environmental factors produce loss of neurones to areas of the brain controlling cognition and leave plaques and tangles as neuropathological markers of this destruction. The actual mechanism of destruction might involve free radical activity. When cell loss is sufficient to exhaust neuronal reserves and compensatory mechanisms, dementia is the result.

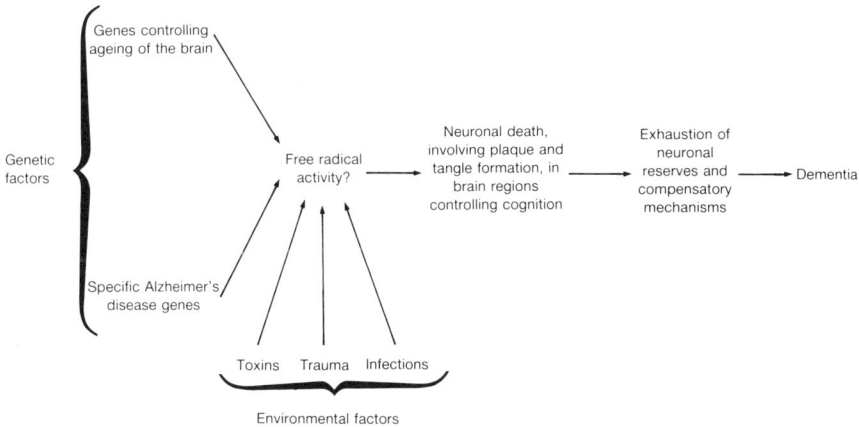

Figure 9.3 Outline of a broad theory of the aetiology of Alzheimer's disease.

While it is not difficult to sketch a broad overarching theory of this sort, it is unfortunately rather jelly-like in its ability to be moulded to fit any new fact. The task ahead is to make specific testable proposals about the genes, toxins, trauma, infections and compensatory mechanisms which could play a role in the aetiology of Alzheimer's disease.

10 Risk factors for vascular dementia

While risk factors for Alzheimer's disease have been the focus of great epidemiological interest over recent years, vascular dementia has not received the same degree of attention. In large part, this neglect may stem from the much lower prevalence of vascular dementia, relative to Alzheimer's disease, in Europe and North America. However, another factor may be the diagnostic uncertainties surrounding vascular dementia. As discussed in Chapter 1, the clinical diagnosis of vascular dementia presents particular difficulties and the classification of types of vascular dementia is still evolving and uncertain.

In 1974, Hachinski, Lassen and Marshall proposed the concept of multi-infarct dementia which, for a decade afterward, came to dominate research on vascular dementia. However, with the advent of CT and MRI scans, the unitary notion of multi-infarct dementia began to break down, with several separate types of vascular dementia being proposed. At the present time there is little agreement about the classification of vascular dementia and the various newly proposed types have had little impact on epidemiological research. For this reason, risk factors for vascular dementia are reviewed here as though it were a unitary disease.

10.1 RISK FACTORS FOR STROKE

If, as stated by Fisher (1968), 'cerebrovascular dementia is a matter of strokes large and small', risk factors for vascular dementia should largely correspond to those for stroke. The correspondence need not, however, be exact. Risk factors for disease to different branches of the vascular tree are not necessarily the same. For example, risk factors for stroke are not identical to those for myocardial infarction, so that populations at increased risk for one are not necessarily at increased risk for the other. Similarly, risk factors for major strokes not resulting in dementia may not be exactly the same as for strokes which do result in dementia. Nevertheless, the overlap is likely to be great and known risk factors for stroke can be regarded as probable risk factors for vascular dementia as well.

The literature on risk factors for stroke is substantial, but has been

Table 10.1   Risk factors for stroke as summarized by the Stroke Council of the American Heart Association

---

Well-documented risk factors

Treatment not feasible or value of treatment not established
  Age and gender
  Familial factors
  Race
  Diabetes mellitus
  Prior stroke
  Asymptomatic carotid bruits
Treatable
  Hypertension
  Cardiac disease
  Transient ischemic attacks
  Elevated hematocrit
  Sickle cell disease

Less well-documented risk factors

Treatment not feasible or value of treatment not established
  Geographic location
  Season and climate
  Socio-economic factors
Treatable but value of treatment not established
  Elevated blood cholesterol and lipids
  Cigarette smoking
  Alcohol consumption
  Oral contraceptive use
  Physical inactivity
  Obesity

---

summarized by a special subcommittee of the Stroke Council of the American Heart Association (Dyken *et al.*, 1984). They classified risk factors as either 'well-documented' or 'less-documented' as shown in Table 10.1 and further subdivided them according to whether or not they are treatable.

A few of these risk factors for stroke could not be meaningfully regarded as risk factors for vascular dementia because they enter into commonly used criteria for clinical diagnosis of the disorder. For example, the widely used Ischemic Score of Hachinski *et al.* (1975) incorporates 'history of strokes' and 'evidence of associated atherosclerosis' as indicators of vascular dementia. Thus, any study which used the Ischemic Score or similar criteria for diagnostic purposes might, *ipso facto*, find that factors such as prior strokes, transient ischemic attacks, cardiac disease and symptomatic carotid bruits are associated with vascular dementia. For this reason, such factors cannot be properly considered as conferring increased risk for vascular dementia unless it is defined independently of them. They are more legitimately seen as indicators that a dementia may be of vascular origin than as risk factors *per se*.

10.2 EVIDENCE OF RISK FACTORS FOR VASCULAR DEMENTIA

Many of the risk factors for stroke in Table 10.1 have also been explicity investigated with vascular dementia. The evidence on these risk factors is reviewed below. Other risk factors mentioned in the table have either not been explicitly investigated for vascular dementia or may be used in its diagnosis. Such factors are not discussed further.

10.2.1 Age and gender

As with Alzheimer's disease, old age is the pre-eminent risk factor for vascular dementia. Studies of the incidence of vascular dementia were reviewed in Chapter 5 and have shown a sharp rise with age suggestive of an exponential increase.

While stroke incidence is higher in males, studies of the incidence of vascular dementia are less clear cut. As summarized in Chapter 5, two studies have found a higher male rate, one a weak trend towards a higher female rate, and a fourth found no sex difference. Studies of prevalence, however, more clearly show a higher rate of vascular dementia in males, as do neuropathological studies of dementia cases.

10.2.2 Familial factors

There is evidence for a familial predisposition to stroke and also for vascular dementia. Åkesson (1969), in his study of a Swedish rural community, observed that both parents and siblings of vascular dementia cases had increased risk for this disorder. Similarly, in a longitudinal study of ageing twins, Jarvik and Matsuyama (1983) found that stroke in a parent increased the risk of both twins of a pair developing a vascular dementia.

10.2.3 Race and geographic location

Japan has a higher incidence of stroke than other developed countries. This increased incidence seems to be due to environmental factors. A study of stroke in Japanese men living in Japan, Hawaii and California found incidence to be quite different in the three locations, being highest in Japan and lowest in California (Kagan *et al.*, 1976). Cerebrovascular disease mortality in Japan has also been found to differ greatly between regions and to be associated with diet. Regions with high intake of certain foods characteristic of the traditional Japanese diet (pork, seaweed, miso, pickled vegetables, soy sauce and salted fish) have higher stroke mortality than regions consuming more characteristically Western foods (wheat, butter and margarine, beef and eggs) (Omura *et al.*, 1987). Unfortunately, no data are available on the incidence of vascular dementia in Japan. However, as discussed in Chapter 4, both prevalence studies and neuropathological studies indicate that vascular dementia is more common than Alzheimer's disease in Japan, in contrast to the situation in Western Europe and North America. These findings indicate that the incidence of vascular dementia is also likely to be high in Japan.

China may also have a higher incidence of vascular dementia. While incidence studies and neuropathological studies are not available, prevalence studies have indicated that vascular dementia is more common than Alzheimer's disease in China. Although Russian prevalence studies have also reported vascular dementia to be more common than Alzheimer's disease, this difference appears to be due to diagnostic fashion. As discussed in Chapter 4, neuropathological studies indicate that Russian psychiatrists over-diagnose vascular dementia at the expense of Alzheimer's disease.

In the United States, stroke mortality is found to be higher in Blacks than in Whites. However, no data exist to say whether Blacks have a correspondingly high incidence of vascular dementia.

10.2.4 Diabetes mellitus

Meyer *et al.* (1988) found diabetes mellitus to be present in 20% of vascular dementia cases compared to only 7% of normal controls and this difference was statistically significant. In a comparison of stroke patients with and without dementia, Ladurner *et al.* (1982) found diabetes in 20% of the demented patients compared to 10% of the non-demented patients. While the magnitude of this difference is similar to that reported by Meyer *et al.* (1988), the effect was not statistically significant.

10.2.5 Hypertension

According to Dyken *et al.* (1984), hypertension is the major risk factor for stroke. However, its role in vascular dementia is difficult to evaluate because the presence of hypertension is often a contributing factor in making a clinical diagnosis of the disorder. Nevertheless, there are some studies in which vascular dementia is diagnosed using neuropathological evidence and diagnostic artefact is not a problem. St Clair and Whalley (1983) divided 88 demented patients into vascular, Alzheimer and mixed groups on neuropathological grounds. The vascular cases were higher than the Alzheimer cases in both systolic and diastolic blood pressure. No vascular dementia case had a systolic pressure below 140 mm Hg, whereas half of the Alzheimer cases had a systolic pressure this low.

A variety of vascular dementia in which hypertension is believed to play a very strong role is Binswanger's disease. Reviewing all published pathologically-verified cases of Binswanger's disease from 1912 to 1986, Babikian and Ropper (1987) found that 98% of those with relevant information available were hypertensive. Although no controls were available, this prevalence is so high as to clearly indicate a role for hypertension in Binswanger's disease.

Another piece of evidence implicating hypertension as a risk factor comes from Ladurner *et al.*'s (1982) study comparing stroke patients with and without dementia. Hypertension was found in 68% of the demented patients compared to only 23% of the non-demented patients. This finding suggests that hypertension is a specific risk factor for vascular dementia over and above its role for stroke in general. Other evidence that hypertension may have an influence on cognitive functioning additional to stroke comes from a large general population survey of elderly people by Wallace *et al.* (1985). They excluded individuals with a history of stroke and found a correlation between hypertension and poor verbal memory which persisted even with statistical adjustment for age, education, self-perceived health status, current alcohol consumption, depressive symptoms, anti-hypertensive medication and physical activity. There are also many clinic-based studies comparing hypertensives and normotensives which show that hypertension is associated with poorer cognitive functioning, even in young and middle-aged adults (Boller *et al.*, 1977; Pentz *et al.*, 1979; Schultz *et al.*, 1979; Franceschi *et al.*, 1982). Whether hypertension has a direct causal effect on cognitive function is, however, unclear. Some evidence for a relationship comes from a longitudinal study of individuals aged 60–69 by Wilkie and Eisdorfer (1971) which showed that hypertension predicted intellectual decline over a ten-year follow-up period. If hypertension directly caused cognitive impairment, we might expect treatment to improve it. However, treated hypertensives still have poor cognitive functioning (Franceschi *et al.*, 1982).

10.2.6 Blood cholesterol

According to Dyken et al. (1984), the contribution of blood cholesterol to stroke is not clear but, if there is an increased risk, it is confined to individuals less than 50 years of age. The situation with vascular dementia similarly lacks clarity. Meyer *et al.* (1988) found no association between hyperlipidaemia and vascular dementia, while Lehtonen and Luutonen (1986) found cholesterol to be higher in vascular dementia cases compared to normals but, surprisingly, not compared to Alzheimer cases. Studies focusing on high density lipoprotein (HDL) cholesterol have, however, found a consistent association, with vascular dementia cases having lowered levels. This association was first reported by Muckle and Roy (1985) in a small study, but has been replicated by Erkinjuntti *et al.* (1985) and Zanetti *et al.* (1985). Muckle and Roy (1985) argued that the association between lowered HDL cholesterol and vascular dementia was so strong as to make this a useful diagnostic test for differentiating this disorder from Alzheimer's disease. However, the other studies reported overlapping distributions between vascular and Alzheimer patients, indicating that HDL cholesterol levels are of limited diagnostic value. The only study not to find lowered HDL cholesterol levels in vascular dementia was by Lehtonen and Luutonen (1986). Their study was confined to patients aged over 90, suggesting the possibility that age is an important moderating variable in the relationship.

10.2.7 Cigarette smoking and alcohol consumption

Dyken *et al.* (1984) have classified these as 'less well-documented' risk factors for stroke. As possible risk factors for vascular dementia they have received little attention. Both Pinessi *et al.* (1983) and Meyer *et al.* (1988) have reported smoking to be more common in vascular dementia cases than in controls. With alcohol consumption, however, Pinessi *et al.* (1983) found an association, but Meyer *et al.* (1988) did not. The lack of association in Meyer *et al.*'s (1988) study could be due to the fact that it excluded heavy drinkers.

10.2.8 Other possible risk factors

One possible risk factor for vascular dementia not included in Table 10.1 is a history of depression. Bucht *et al.* (1984) found this to be a factor in 30% of vascular dementia patients compared to only 5% of Alzheimer patients and 0% of controls. By contrast, the same study found that *current* signs of depression were more common in Alzheimer's disease than in vascular dementia. This factor merits further investigation.

10.3 CONCLUSION

The limited available evidence on risk factors for vascular dementia is generally consistent with what is known about risk factors for stroke. However, several of the risk factors for stroke listed in Table 10.1 have not been specifically investigated as risk factors for vascular dementia. Although the risk factors for stroke and vascular dementia may be broadly the same, the relative importance of risk factors for strokes which result in dementia may be somewhat different than for strokes which do not. Furthermore, the importance of various risk factors may be found to vary between types of vascular dementia once the confusion over their classification is resolved.

11 *Prospects for prevention*

The ultimate purpose of investigating the epidemiology of a disorder is to promote its prevention. In order to prevent a disorder it is desirable to understand its aetiology. However, even without a full understanding of aetiology, prevention can be carried out through modification of risk factors. This strategy is limited, however, by the fact that some risk factors are, by their nature, not modifiable (e.g. family history of a disease, fingerprint patterns). Furthermore, a risk factor is, strictly speaking, only a correlate of disease incidence. If the association between the risk factor and the disease is not a causal one then modification of the risk factor would have no effect. Because the aetiology of neither Alzheimer's disease nor vascular dementia is understood, the strategy of modifying risk factors is presently the most viable option for prevention. If this strategy was applied, what benefits might reasonably be expected? In answering this question, it is useful to consider first the degree to which chronic diseases of ageing are in general preventable.

11.1 AGE-RELATED AND AGE-DEPENDENT DISEASES

Brody and Schneider (1986) have drawn a very useful distinction between **age-dependent** and **age-related** diseases. Age-dependent diseases are those in which the pathology is an intrinsic part of the ageing process. Age-related diseases, on the other hand, vary in incidence with age, but are not necessarily related to the ageing process. For an age-dependent disease, incidence and mortality rise exponentially with age, while for an age-related disease the occurrence may increase with age and then decrease or may continue to increase in a less than exponential manner.

This distinction has important implications for prevention. Age-related diseases can be successfully prevented if an individual can negotiate the period of life where there is maximal risk without exposure to aetiological agents. By contrast, age-dependent diseases cannot be completely prevented. They can be postponed through modifying environmental risk factors, but their eventual occurrence is inevitable. If an individual can postpone the onset of an age-dependent disease so that death from another cause intervenes, then the disease can be

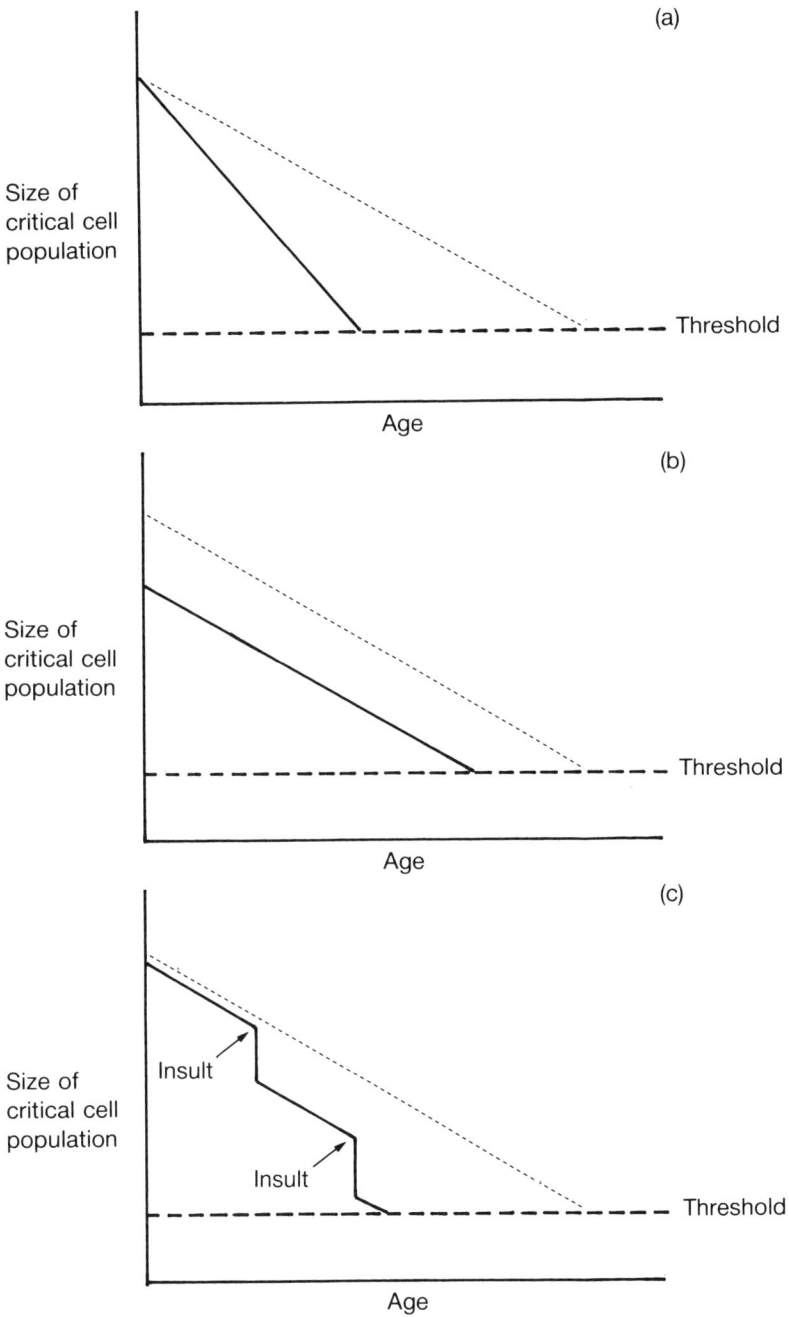

Figure 11.1 A model of age-dependent chronic diseases. Adapted from Brody and Schneider (1986).

regarded as 'prevented'. Age-dependent diseases become increasingly common in a population as premature causes of death, like infectious diseases and accidents, are eliminated. They reflect the physiological processes which underlie the finite human lifespan. Age-dependent diseases can be substituted for each other as causes of death, but cannot be avoided altogether. Thus, as mortality due to one age-dependent disease is reduced, the importance of others must correspondingly increase.

Brody and Schneider (1986) have provided a useful model of age-dependent chronic diseases which illustrates the way in which risk can vary between individuals and be postponed by preventive measures. According to this model, ageing is associated with loss of either cell numbers or cell function from particular populations of cells. When this cell loss reaches a critical threshold in a population, the individual becomes susceptible to an age-dependent disease. Figure 11.1 illustrates the model. Individuals may differ in the rate of cell loss (as in Figure 11.1a) or could be born with a small functioning cell population (as in Figure 11.1b). Either of these situations would result in individual differences in age of disease onset. Genetic factors are likely to act in either of these manners. Environmental insults will also produce loss of cells (shown in Figure 11.1c) and so reduce the age of onset. Preventive programmes might reduce the frequency of these insults and so delay disease onset.

In discussing the prevention of Alzheimer's disease and vascular dementia it is useful to consider whether they could be age-dependent diseases. Importantly, the occurrence of both is known to increase markedly with age. Prevalence increases in an exponential manner, and what is known about incidence is also consistent with an exponential increase. In this respect, both Alzheimer's disease and vascular dementia fulfill the criteria for age-dependent diseases. However, in the case of Alzheimer's disease there is some disagreement about whether it is intrinsic to the ageing process. Creasey and Rapoport (1985), for example, regard Alzheimer's disease as a pathology superimposed on the ageing brain and claim that it differs in a number of ways from accelerated ageing. Others, like Brayne and Calloway (1988) and Storandt *et al.* (1988) have argued that there are no qualitative features which distinguish normal brain ageing from Alzheimer's disease and that they are different points on a continuum.

Different views of Alzheimer's disease as an age-dependent or age-related disease are also implied by the theories reviewed in Chapter 9. Under an autosomal dominant, toxic-exposure or infectious-agent theory, it would be an age-related disease. Alzheimer's disease could be completely prevented by avoiding the toxic exposure or infectious agent or blocking the expression of the responsible gene. By contrast, an ageing–environment interaction theory would imply that it is an age-dependent disease that could be postponed but not completely prevented. Whether Alzheimer's disease is age-dependent or age-related cannot therefore be decided at this point in time, but the possibility that it can only be delayed, rather than completely avoided, must be given strong consideration.

11.2 PREVENTION OF ALZHEIMER'S DISEASE BY RISK FACTOR MODIFICATION

Given that the aetiology of Alzheimer's disease is far from understood and that various aetiological theories have conflicting implications for prevention, the strategy of modifying risk factors seems the most feasible way ahead. Unfortunately, very few of the risk factors reviewed in Chapter 8 are susceptible to modification. Of the risk factors assessed as 'confirmed' or 'possible', only one – head trauma – is readily modifiable. Assuming that this factor is indeed causally associated with Alzheimer's disease, what would be the effect on disease incidence if it could be eliminated?

The benefit to public health of eliminating an exposure can be summarized by the **aetiologic fraction** (Schlesselman, 1982). This gives the proportion of all cases in a population which can be attributed to the exposure. To calculate the aetiologic fraction it is necessary to know the relative risk associated with the exposure and the proportion of the population exposed to it. In his meta-analysis of eight case-control studies, Mortimer (1989) calculated an odds ratio of 2.77 for exposure to head trauma. This odds ratio can be used as an approximation to the relative risk of exposure. The proportion of the population exposed to head trauma can be estimated from the proportion of controls with a history of head trauma in the same case-control studies. From the seven studies reporting these data, exposure to head trauma varied from a low of 1.8% to a high of 14.6%, with 3.8% being the median. Obviously, the frequency of head trauma varies considerably depending on the definition used in a study. Taking the most conservative estimate to calculate the aetiologic fraction, it can be estimated that 3% of Alzheimer's disease cases are attributable to head trauma. Taking the median estimate of exposure to head trauma gives a figure of 6% of cases attributable to this exposure. Although these are small percentages, they may refer to a large number of cases, since Alzheimer's disease is not an uncommon disorder. Therefore, the elimination of head trauma would, assuming it is a true risk factor, have a noticeable public health impact. The complete elimination of head trauma may not be a feasible goal, but even a substantial reduction might be worth pursuing. However, this is a goal already being pursued in many countries through measures such as legislation for the compulsory wearing of seat-belts and encouragement to wear helmets during high-risk activities.

The evaluation of efforts at risk factor modification poses particular challenges. In some instances, there could be decades intervening between an environmental exposure and disease onset. Attempts to evaluate the removal of such an exposure would be demanding in both time and resources. There is a need for studies which monitor the incidence of Alzheimer's disease over time. It is a sobering thought that the incidence of Alzheimer's disease could currently be either falling or rising in certain parts of the world and we probably would not know. The short-cut solution, which works satisfactorily for many diseases, is to monitor disease mortality using death certificate data. However, the validity of death certificate data on Alzheimer's disease is currently too weak to make this a path worth pursuing.

11.3 PREVENTION OF VASCULAR DEMENTIA BY RISK FACTOR MODIFICATION

At the present state of knowledge, vascular dementia has more modifiable risk factors than Alzheimer's disease and so presents greater possibility for preventive action. Indeed, there is evidence from both the United States and Japan that the incidence of stroke has been declining over recent decades (Garraway *et al.*, 1979; Ueda *et al.*, 1981). In addition, stroke mortality, as assessed from death certificates, has declined in many developed countries. Whether this decline in stroke occurrence is due to deliberate preventive actions, such as the control of hypertension, or whether it is a fortuitous effect of changing lifestyle is unknown. This reduction in stroke incidence might be expected to have a corresponding effect on vascular dementia. However, the only existing data on the subject, from the Lundby study in Sweden (Rorsman *et al.*, 1986), found no significant change in incidence of vascular dementia between 1947–1957 and 1957–1972.

Although there is substantial knowledge about risk factors for stroke, there have not been controlled studies of the effects of risk factor modification on the incidence of vascular dementia. There is, however, one uncontrolled study of risk factor modification in patients already suffering from vascular dementia. This is a study of secondary rather than primary prevention. Meyer *et al.* (1986) studied 52 vascular dementia patients over periods ranging from 3 to 48 months. Cognitive performance was monitored every three months and compared with that in Alzheimer's disease patients and normal volunteers. Vascular patients who had hypertension were treated with medication while smokers were counselled to give up the habit. The outcome was quite variable in those treated for hypertension, with some showing improved cognition and others declining. By contrast, the Alzheimer's disease patients showed a more consistent trend towards cognitive decline and the normals remained relatively stable. The treated hypertensives who declined were found to have a mean treated systolic blood pressure of 128 mm Hg, as against a mean of 137 mm Hg for those who improved. Meyer *et al.* (1986) argued that there is an optimal window for systolic blood pressure between 135 and 150 mm Hg and that lower pressure than this could cause deterioration. Giving up smoking appeared to have benefits because those normotensive patients who gave up the habit showed significantly improved cognitive performance compared to those who continued. Control of other risk factors, including diabetes, hyperlipidaemia and alcohol consumption, did not affect cognitive performance in this study.

11.4 PREVENTIVE EFFECTS OF ANTIPLATELET TREATMENT

An alternative approach to prevention is the use of medications which alter processes associated with the disease. Use of antiplatelet treatment to prevent vascular diseases has been the focus of a number of important studies. In Britain, Peto *et al.* (1988) have reported on a randomized trial of prophylactic daily aspirin in over 5000 healthy male physicians. Over a six-year period, there was no significant difference in incidence of either fatal or non-fatal vascular diseases. In fact, the incidence of disabling stroke was marginally higher in the group receiving aspirin. A similar preventive study has been carried out with over 20 000 American male physicians using a randomized double-blind placebo-controlled design (Steering Committee of the Physicians' Health Study Research Group, 1989). Over a follow-up period averaging five years, the incidence of myocardial infarction was significantly reduced, but stroke had a non-significantly higher incidence. The results of these studies indicate no benefit of using aspirin for the primary prevention of stroke and, by implication, vascular dementia.

Rather different results emerge, however, when antiplatelet treatment is used for secondary prevention of stroke in individuals with a history of vascular disease (Antiplatelet Trialists' Collaboration, 1988). A meta-analysis of 25 randomized trials of such treatment found that non-fatal strokes were reduced by a quarter and vascular deaths (due to stroke of myocardial infarction) by a sixth. This meta-analysis covered several different treatments (aspirin, sulphinpyrazone, aspirin plus dipyridamole), but no difference was found between them in effectiveness. Furthermore, different doses of aspirin were used in various studies (300–325 mg vs. 900–1500 mg), but this had no effect on outcome. The authors therefore concluded that: 'For the present the least expensive and most convenient antiplatelet treatment appears to be aspirin, perhaps at a dose no greater than (or even much less than) 300–325 mg/day.' (p. 329). It could reasonably be presumed that antiplatelet treatment might have a similar secondary preventive effect with vascular dementia. Indeed, small trials by Kellett (1988) and Meyer *et al.* (1989) indicate that this is so. Kellett (1988) carried out a double-blind crossover comparison of aspirin, cyclandelate (a peripheral vasodilator) and placebo with 31 patients suffering from vascular dementia. Patients received each of the treatments for six months. It was found that both active treatments were significantly better than placebo in preventing further vascular incidents. In the Meyer *et al.* (1989) study, cases of vascular dementia were randomly assigned either daily aspirin or no treatment. Yearly follow-ups for up to three years showed that the 37 treated patients did significantly better than the 33 controls in both cognitive performance and cerebral blood flow.

The above studies show that the use of antiplatelet treatment for secondary prevention of vascular dementia may be feasible. However, the widespread use of such treatment might have the effect of improving survival in cases of vascular dementia, thereby increasing the prevalence of this disorder. There is a need to evaluate whether improved survival in vascular dementia also implies improved quality of life. If antiplatelet treatment led to more years of cognitively- and physically-impaired existence, one might question its overall benefits to the patient and to the community.

11.5 CONCLUSION

With the ageing of the world's population, the prevalence of dementing disorders is expected to increase greatly, placing increasing strains on national health and welfare budgets. While the development of success-ful treatments for these disorders might eventually slow their progression, or even partially restore lost function, prevention remains the ultimate hope. If Alzheimer's disease and vascular dementia turn out to be diseases superimposed on the ageing process, then it is a real possiblity that these diseases can one day be eliminated from the aged population. However, if they are an intrinsic part of human ageing, elimination of these disorders will not be feasible, unless some means is found to alter the very processes of ageing. When all the avoidable causes of death are eliminated, there remains the fundamental ageing of the human body which will eventually lead to the failure of some critical organ system such as the brain. If, for example, Alzheimer's disease turns out to be the age-dependent failure of certain brain processes, then the appropriate public health goal must be to delay onset and thereby prolong the duration of healthy old age. While delaying onset would increase human welfare by providing a longer lifespan, the burden of terminal dementing diseases would still exist as before. Whether or not Alzheimer's disease and vascular dementia are intrinsic parts of the ageing process is presently unknown and will only be resolved with a greater understanding of ageing in general. In the meantime, it is uncertain whether elimination of disease or its postponement is the more realistic goal for preventive action.

However, whatever the goal of prevention, the immediately feasible path ahead is to pursue modification of risk factors. Therefore, the search for modifiable risk factors must be a key focus for epidemiological research on dementing disorders. As far as Alzheimer's disease is concerned, the results of this search have been rather disappointing so far. However, as the first case-control study of risk factors for Alzheimer's disease was only published in 1982, the search is still in its infancy. The current situation with vascular dementia is, by contrast, more optimistic, even though it has received less epidemiological attention than Alzheimer's disease. There are several possible risk factors for vascular dementia which are potentially modifiable, providing a useful focus for preventive action. Indeed, the reduction in stroke incidence which has been reported over recent decades clearly demonstrates that chronic diseases of ageing are preventable, and augurs well for the preventability of vascular dementia in particular.

In recent years, there have been exciting developments from basic biomedical research on dementing disorders, particularly Alzheimer's disease. Both the general public and the research community see this type of research as providing the breakthroughs which will be translated into cures. By contrast, epidemiological research has produced no headline-grabbing findings and promises no easy cures. Yet, in the history of disease control, preventive efforts have arguably contributed much more to the prolongation of human life than has clinical medicine, and it is epidemiology which underpins these efforts. For all we know, it may be epidemiology which eventually provides the foundation for the successful control of Alzheimer's disease and related disorders.

Appendix A *DSM-III-R Diagnostic Criteria. From American Psychiatric Association (1987)*

DIAGNOSTIC CRITERIA FOR DEMENTIA

1. Demonstrable evidence of impairment in short- and long-term memory. Impairment in short-term memory (inability to learn new information) may be indicated by inability to remember three objects after five minutes. Long-term memory impairment (inability to remember information that was known in the past) may be indicated by inability to remember past personal information (e.g. what happened yesterday, birthplace, occupation) or facts of common knowledge (e.g. past Presidents' well-known dates).
2. At least one of the following:
   (a) impairment in abstract thinking, as indicated by inability to find similarities and differences between related words, difficulty in defining words and concepts, and other similar tasks;
   (b) impaired judgment, as indicated by inability to make reasonable plans to deal with interpersonal, family, and job-related problems and issues;
   (c) other disturbances of higher cortical function, such as aphasia (disorder of language), apraxia (inability to carry out motor activities despite intact comprehension and motor function), agnosia (failure to recognize or identify objects despite intact sensory function), and 'constructional difficulty' (e.g. inability to copy three-dimensional figures, assemble blocks, or arrange sticks in specific designs);
   (d) personality change, i.e. alteration or accentuation of premorbid traits.
3. The disturbance in (1) and (2) significantly interferes with work or usual social activities or relationships with others.
4. Not occurring exclusively during the course of delirium.
5. Either (a) or (b):
   (a) there is evidence from the history, physical examination, or laboratory tests of a specific organic factor (or factors) judged to be etiologically related to the disturbance;

(b) in the absence of such evidence, an etiological organic factor can be presumed if the disturbance cannot be accounted for by any non-organic mental disorder, e.g. major depression accounting for cognitive impairment.

CRITERIA FOR SEVERITY OF DEMENTIA

Mild Although work or social activities are significantly impaired, the capacity for independent living remains, with adequate personal hygiene and relatively intact judgment.

Moderate Independent living is hazardous, and some degree of supervision is necessary.

Severe Activities of daily living are so impaired that continual supervision is required, e.g. unable to maintain minimal personal hygiene; largely incoherent or mute.

DIAGNOSTIC CRITERIA FOR PRIMARY DEGENERATIVE DEMENTIA OF THE ALZHEIMER TYPE

1. Dementia.
2. Insidious onset with a generally progressive deteriorating course.
3. Exclusion of all other specific causes of dementia by history, physical examination, and laboratory tests.

DIAGNOSTIC CRITERIA FOR MULTI-INFARCT DEMENTIA

1. Dementia.
2. Stepwise deteriorating course with 'patchy' distribution of deficits (i.e. affecting some functions, but not others) early in the course.
3. Focal neurological signs and symptoms (e.g. exaggeration of deep tendon reflexes, extensor plantar response, pseudobulbar palsy, gait abnormalities, weakness of an extremity, etc.).
4. Evidence from history, physical examination, or laboratory tests of significant cerebrovascular disease (recorded on Axis III) that is judged to be etiologically related to the disturbance.

Appendix B *NINCDS–ADRDA criteria for clinical diagnosis of Alzheimer's disease. From McKhann et al. (1984)*

1. The criteria for the clinical diagnosis of *probable* Alzheimer's disease include:

    dementia established by clinical examination and documented by the Mini-Mental Test, Blessed Dementia Scale, or some similar examination, and confirmed by neuropsychological tests;

    deficits in two or more areas of cognition;

    progressive worsening of memory and other cognitive functions;

    no disturbance of consciousness;

    onset between ages 40 and 90, most often after age 65; and

    absence of systemic disorders or other brain diseases that in and of themselves could account for the progressive deficits in memory and cognition.

2. The diagnosis of *probable* Alzheimer's disease is supported by:

    progressive deterioration of specific cognitive functions such as language (aphasia), motor skills (apraxia), and perception (agnosia);

    impaired activities of daily living and altered patterns of behaviour;

    family history of similar disorders particularly if confirmed neuropathologically; and

    laboratory results of:

    normal lumbar puncture as evaluated by standard techniques.

    normal pattern of non-specific changes in EEG, such as increased slow-wave activity, and

    evidence of cerebral atrophy on CT with progression documented by serial observation.

3. Other clinical features consistent with the diagnosis of *probable* Alzheimer's disease, after exclusion of causes of dementia other than Alzheimer's disease, include:

    plateaus in the course of progression of the illness;

    associated symptoms of depression, insomnia, incontinence,

delusion, illusions, hallucinations, catastrophic verbal, emotional, or physical outbursts, sexual disorders, and weight loss;

other neurological abnormalities in some patients, especially with more advanced disease and including motor signs such as increased muscle tone, myoclonus, or gait disorder;

seizures in advanced disease; and

CT normal for age.

4. Features that make the diagnosis of *probable* Alzheimer's disease uncertain or unlikely include:

sudden, apoplectic onset;

focal neurological findings such as hemiparesis, sensory loss, visual field deficits, and inco-ordination early in the course of the illness; and

seizures or gait disturbances at the onset or very early in the course of the illness.

5. Clinical diagnosis of *possible* Alzheimer's disease:

may be made on the basis of the dementia syndrome, in the absence of other neurological, psychiatric, or systemic disorders sufficient to cause dementia, and in the presence of variations in the onset, in the presentation, or in the clinical course;

may be made in the presence of a second systemic or brain disorder sufficient to produce dementia, which is not considered to be the cause of the dementia; and

should be used in research studies when a single, gradually progressive severe cognitive deficit is identified in the absence of other identifiable cause.

6. Criteria for diagnosis of *definite* Alzheimer's disease are:

the clinical criteria for probable Alzheimer's disease and histopathological evidence obtained from a biopsy or autopsy.

7. Classification of Alzheimer's disease for research purposes should specify features that may differentiate subtypes of the disorder, such as:

familial occurrence;

onset before age of 65;

presence of trisomy-21; and

coexistence of other relevant conditions such as Parkinson's disease.

Appendix C Projected increases in population and in the number of dementia cases for 29 developed countries

	Population (thousands) 1980	Percentage increase over 1980 value in year:								
		1985	1990	1995	2000	2005	2010	2015	2020	2025
Australia										
Total population	14 695	6.83	13.70	20.40	26.76	32.67	38.27	43.76	48.95	53.62
Population ⩾60	2 016	12.95	25.06	33.10	41.79	54.99	76.08	98.71	122.60	145.00
Dementia cases	–	12.94	28.69	44.59	59.20	73.42	87.97	105.30	130.30	161.90
Austria										
Total population	7 505	−0.04	0.03	0.15	0.16	−0.29	−0.79	−1.28	−1.94	−3.01
Population ⩾60	1 443	2.91	4.09	3.40	6.87	12.76	17.34	21.57	28.92	39.04
Dementia cases	–	4.22	5.88	4.83	6.29	12.44	15.80	19.97	27.21	35.26
Belgium										
Total population	9 852	0.52	0.99	1.22	1.61	1.69	1.84	1.97	2.05	2.05
Population ⩾60	1 803	5.50	9.99	13.99	16.21	16.55	23.76	31.76	41.20	50.19
Dementia cases	–	4.96	8.00	10.58	14.47	22.38	27.46	31.32	37.35	45.59

Bulgaria										
Total population	8 862	2.36	4.33	5.98	7.59	8.89	10.13	11.33	12.53	13.63
Population ≥60	1 388	12.82	24.50	34.44	38.83	40.63	48.05	53.75	58.07	61.17
Dementia cases	–	11.66	22.61	32.82	44.76	60.67	71.01	78.03	83.63	92.34
Canada										
Total population	24 090	5.55	11.03	15.89	20.08	23.84	27.60	31.40	35.01	38.07
Population ≥60	3 305	14.16	25.89	34.88	43.53	57.71	80.91	109.10	133.50	156.40
Dementia	–	15.51	32.27	48.71	64.02	79.39	94.72	113.30	139.50	173.30
Czechoslovakia										
Total population	15 311	1.75	3.38	5.51	8.30	10.87	13.04	14.97	16.92	18.59
Population ≥60	2 405	5.61	9.06	11.60	13.01	19.00	33.10	48.57	57.87	62.25
Dementia cases	–	5.05	7.32	8.08	11.99	21.46	29.03	37.96	50.59	67.17
Denmark										
Total population	5 123	−0.02	−0.06	−0.31	−0.80	−1.74	−3.01	−4.53	−6.31	−8.45
Population ≥60	998	3.31	3.71	3.01	4.41	12.22	23.15	29.76	34.67	39.88
Dementia cases	–	6.83	12.08	15.00	17.08	19.72	23.14	29.64	39.54	50.86
Finland										
Total population	4 780	2.32	3.89	5.00	5.75	6.09	6.11	5.92	5.40	4.48
Population ≥60	782	7.68	14.34	18.31	22.92	29.96	49.30	62.87	71.70	79.00
Dementia cases	–	13.86	25.12	33.36	40.55	49.94	60.06	70.77	85.86	104.70
France										
Total population	53 714	1.69	3.28	4.89	6.42	7.27	7.85	8.27	8.63	8.78
Population ≥60	9 242	4.46	9.84	16.13	20.21	21.55	33.91	44.89	54.72	63.73
Dementia cases	–	0.26	−0.75	−0.09	3.63	12.58	19.21	24.58	31.24	42.39
German Democratic Republic										
Total population	16 737	0.18	0.91	1.57	2.47	3.26	4.15	4.77	4.93	4.98
Population ≥60	3 214	−5.70	−6.85	−3.43	8.69	15.22	13.48	21.67	28.42	37.80
Dementia cases	–	−3.38	−8.77	−13.80	−12.49	−4.70	7.22	11.64	18.33	22.13

	Population (thousands) 1980	Percentage increase over 1980 value in year:								
		1985	1990	1995	2000	2005	2010	2015	2020	2025
Germany, Federal Republic										
Total population	61 566	−1.12	−2.00	−2.57	−3.38	−5.05	−7.09	−9.17	−11.22	−13.12
Population ⩾60	11 888	2.53	5.22	8.40	11.94	24.83	28.38	28.38	32.12	40.01
Dementia cases	–	5.74	7.92	7.64	11.25	19.77	26.16	32.63	38.42	40.73
Great Britain										
Total population	55 945	0.32	0.44	0.65	0.73	0.51	0.33	0.29	0.24	−0.05
Population ⩾60	11 271	3.21	3.09	1.77	1.65	3.06	10.25	14.27	19.70	27.60
Dementia cases	–	6.83	11.27	13.22	14.40	16.05	17.25	19.76	25.25	33.50
Greece										
Total population	9 643	2.44	4.57	6.51	8.23	9.55	10.37	10.93	11.41	11.88
Population ⩾60	1 683	4.64	15.69	26.80	34.76	36.24	40.40	42.42	46.64	52.70
Dementia cases	–	9.33	18.33	26.40	34.83	46.56	59.04	65.44	67.78	70.73
Hungary										
Total population	10 711	−0.13	−0.49	−0.47	0.03	0.17	−0.07	−0.46	−0.75	−1.06
Population ⩾60	1 841	5.87	10.44	13.87	16.15	19.41	24.96	36.32	41.98	39.64
Dementia cases	–	3.84	7.09	9.94	15.05	24.29	30.02	36.29	43.94	52.40
Ireland										
Total population	3 401	6.09	13.00	20.05	27.02	33.61	39.39	45.96	51.63	56.60
Population ⩾60	505	3.18	3.37	3.77	5.95	10.71	23.21	37.90	55.56	79.96
Dementia cases	–	3.91	8.44	12.57	17.28	20.91	26.26	35.61	49.91	71.24
Italy										
Total population	57 070	0.40	0.86	1.79	2.76	2.92	2.39	1.55	0.76	0.19
Population ⩾60	9 846	8.49	16.06	22.58	30.55	33.00	39.53	42.95	47.45	55.87
Dementia cases	–	8.93	17.04	23.15	30.57	42.03	50.25	56.40	61.92	68.09

Japan											
Total population	116 807	3.37	6.04	8.54	11.06	13.05	13.90	13.91	13.53	13.08
Population ≥60	15 021	16.38	37.99	60.71	80.64	100.40	124.00	132.87	131.00	128.30
Dementia cases	–	20.57	42.96	67.19	93.27	125.90	154.70	180.20	199.70	215.40
Netherlands											
Total population	14 150	2.47	4.23	5.72	6.59	6.70	6.41	5.85	5.02	3.82
Population ≥60	2 222	7.47	14.09	19.94	26.42	35.73	54.95	70.21	85.10	99.01
Dementia cases	–	6.00	14.04	21.41	29.48	38.81	49.98	61.63	78.54	99.50
New Zealand											
Total population	3 169	4.70	9.31	13.95	18.30	22.03	25.21	28.12	30.64	32.60
Population ≥60	445	8.78	16.44	20.05	26.80	36.49	55.18	72.75	94.37	118.70
Dementia cases	–	10.16	23.12	34.06	43.40	52.86	64.28	77.84	98.68	125.60
Norway											
Total population	4 086	1.37	2.23	2.81	3.16	3.30	3.50	3.84	4.21	4.28
Population ≥60	828	5.07	5.79	2.77	0.00	2.65	12.91	22.20	31.60	39.20
Dementia cases	–	7.48	14.56	19.57	21.20	20.83	19.83	22.60	31.79	45.33
Poland											
Total population	35 574	4.53	8.26	11.46	14.74	17.90	20.71	23.18	25.34	27.30
Population ≥60	4 696	9.44	21.90	33.61	42.58	43.73	59.64	84.60	107.00	116.00
Dementia cases	–	10.38	18.90	26.45	38.26	54.52	69.23	82.65	97.71	118.10
Portugal											
Total population	9 884	3.32	6.66	10.18	13.43	16.27	18.80	21.08	23.13	24.79
Population ≥60	1 442	7.62	16.29	23.98	29.18	32.02	40.75	54.47	70.41	82.26
Dementia cases	–	9.08	19.29	29.40	41.20	53.36	64.26	74.53	86.31	104.10
Romania											
Total population	22 201	3.68	7.27	11.21	15.18	18.74	21.94	25.11	28.35	31.74
Population ≥60	2 942	11.18	25.08	39.50	53.67	55.23	61.05	73.96	85.32	86.98
Dementia cases	–	10.57	19.92	29.18	43.65	64.07	80.14	92.72	102.30	111.60

	Population (thousands) 1980	Percentage increase over 1980 value in year: 1985	1990	1995	2000	2005	2010	2015	2020	2025
Spain										
Total population	37 430	2.97	6.19	9.56	12.84	15.71	17.91	19.64	21.25	22.85
Population ≥60	5 565	8.86	20.00	32.17	40.40	42.82	48.98	55.33	66.06	80.97
Dementia cases	–	11.75	23.86	36.22	49.14	62.84	75.33	83.87	90.26	100.00
Sweden										
Total population	8 310	0.49	−0.06	−0.84	−1.73	−2.78	−3.73	−4.73	−5.90	−7.26
Population ≥60	1 824	4.28	3.89	1.54	0.55	6.03	15.03	19.14	21.06	22.87
Dementia cases	–	8.27	14.30	17.43	18.52	19.21	19.85	23.21	30.51	39.21
Switzerland										
Total population	6 327	0.74	0.95	0.87	0.22	−1.06	−2.64	−4.42	−6.43	−8.58
Population ≥60	1 154	5.97	11.16	16.96	23.27	32.96	43.43	49.22	53.57	58.39
Dementia cases	–	8.71	14.88	19.47	25.34	33.95	42.67	51.83	61.52	71.03
USA										
Total population	227 738	4.52	9.09	13.57	17.78	21.71	25.71	29.79	33.64	36.97
Population ≥60	35 849	8.19	14.01	16.33	19.39	27.12	37.78	63.63	86.67	105.10
Dementia cases	–	7.59	16.91	25.74	33.47	40.03	45.45	56.75	74.74	99.38
USSR										
Total population	265 493	4.94	9.92	14.32	18.55	22.79	26.98	31.14	34.88	38.70
Population ≥60	34 711	5.35	25.44	37.01	58.81	58.74	63.22	78.92	99.64	119.20
Dementia cases	–	7.90	18.76	28.59	42.90	62.89	82.06	94.75	106.78	116.90
Yugoslavia										
Total population	22 299	3.83	7.16	10.25	13.04	15.25	16.83	18.01	19.02	19.99
Population ≥60	2 575	13.63	34.01	56.48	74.50	80.43	92.51	113.40	129.90	143.10
Dementia cases	–	14.92	28.46	43.42	63.32	92.38	117.70	137.80	153.00	171.30

References

Abalan, F. (1984) Alzheimer's disease and malnutrition: a new etiological hypothesis. *Med. Hypotheses*, **15**, 385–93.

Abalan, F., Achminov, A. and Pinsolle, M. (1985) Malnutrition and Alzheimer's dementia. *Br. J. Psychiatry*, **147**, 320–1.

Adelstein, A.M., Downham, D.Y., Stein, Z. and Susser, M.W. (1968) The epidemiology of mental illness in an English city. *Soc. Psychiatry*, **3**, 47–59.

Aho, K., Harmsen, P., Hatano, S. *et al.* (1980) Cerebrovascular disease in the community: Results of a WHO collaborative study. *Bull. WHO*, **58**, 113–30.

Åkesson, H.O. (1969) A population study of senile and arteriosclerotic psychoses. *Hum. Hered.*, **19**, 546–66.

Amaducci, L.A. Fratiglioni, L., Rocca, W.A. *et al.* (1986) Risk factors for clinically diagnosed Alzheimer's disease: A case-control study of an Italian population. *Neurology*, **36**, 922–31.

American Psychiatric Association (1987) *Diagnostic and Statistical Manual of Mental Disorders*, 3rd edn (revised), American Psychiatric Association, Washington DC.

Amster, L.E. and Krauss, H.H. (1974) The relationship between life crises and mental deterioration in old age. *Int. J. Aging Hum. Dev.*, **5**, 51–5.

Anneren, G., Gardner, A. and Lundin, T. (1986) Increased glutathione peroxidase activity in erythrocytes in patients with Alzheimer's disease/senile dementia of Alzheimer's type. *Acta Neurol. Scand.*, **73**, 86–9.

Anthony, J.C. (1988) The epidemiologic case-control strategy, with applications in psychiatric research, in *Handbook of Social Psychiatry* (eds A.S. Henderson and G. Burrows), Elsevier, Amsterdam.

Anthony, J.C., Niaz, U., LeResche, L.A. *et al.* (1982) Limits of the 'Mini-Mental State' as a screening test for dementia and delirium among hospital patients. *Psychol. Med.*, **12**, 397–408.

Antiplatelet Trialists' Collaboration (1988) Secondary prevention of vascular disease by prolonged antiplatelet treatment. *Br. Med. J.*, **296**, 320–31.

Aubert, R., Parker, R., Rothenburg, R. and May, D. (1987) Methodologic issues in the reported prevalence of Alzheimer's disease on death certificates, in *Proceedings of the 1987 Public Health Conference on Records and Statistics*, US Department of Health and Human Services, Hyatts-ville, Maryland.

Axelson, O., Hane, M. and Hogstedt, C. (1976) A case-reference study on neuropsychiatric disorders among workers exposed to solvents. *Scand. J. Work Environ. Health*, **2**, 14–20.

Babikian, V. and Ropper, A.H. (1987) Binswanger's disease: A review. *Stroke*, **18**, 2–12.

Bachman, D.L., Wolf, P.A., Linn, R.T. *et al.* (1986) Dementia in a community: Prevalence of dementia in the Framingham Heart Study cohort. *Neurology*, **36** (suppl. 1), 107.

Ball, M.J. (1982) Limbic predilection in Alzheimer dementia: Is reactivated herpesvirus involved? *Can. J. Neurol. Sci.*, **9**, 303–6.

Barclay, L.L., Kheyfets, S., Zemcov, A. *et al.* (1985c) Risk factors in Alzheimer's disease, in *Alzheimer's and Parkinson's Diseases* (eds A. Fisher, I. Hanin and C. Lachman), Plenum, New York.

Barclay, L.L., Zemcov, A., Blass, J.P. and McDowell, F.H. (1985a) Factors associated with duration of survival in Alzheimer's disease. *Biol. Psychiatry*, **20**, 86–93.

Barclay, L.L., Zemcov, A., Blass, J.P. and Sansone, J. (1985b) Survival in Alzheimer's disease and vascular dementias. *Neurology*, **35**, 834–40.

Becker, J.T., Huff, F.J., Nebes, R.D. *et al.* (1988) Neuropsychological function in Alzheimer's disease: Pattern of impairment and rates of progression. *Arch, Neurol.*, **45**, 263–8.

Ben-Arie, O., Swartz, L., Teggin, A.F. and Elk, R. (1983) The coloured elderly in Cape Town. A psychosocial, psychiatric and medical community survey. *South African Med. J.*, **64**, 1056–61.

Bentsen, B.G. (1970) *Illness and General Practice*. Universitetsforlaget, Oslo.

Berg, L. (1988) Mild senile dementia of the Alzheimer type: Diagnostic criteria and natural history. *Mount Sinai J. Med.*, **55**, 87–96.

Berg, L., Danziger, W.L., Storandt, M. *et al.* (1984) Predictive features in mild senile dementia of the Alzheimer type. *Neurology*, **34**, 563–9.

Bergmann, K. (1977) Prognosis in chronic brain failure. *Age Ageing*, **6** (suppl.), 61–6.

Bergmann, K., Kay, D.W.K., Foster, E.M. *et al.* (1971) A follow-up study of randomly selected community residents to assess the effects of chronic brain syndrome and cerebrovascular disease. *Psychiatry, Part II; Excerpta Medica Congress Series*, **274**, 856–65.

Berkman, L.F. (1986) The association between educational attainment and mental status examinations: Of etiologic significance for senile dementias or not? *J. Chronic Dis.*, **39**, 171–4.

Berry, P., Groeneweg, G., Gibson, D. and Brown, R.I. (1984) Mental development of adults with Down syndrome. *Am. J. Ment. Defic.*, **89**, 252–6.

Beyreuther, K., Beer, J., Hilbich, C. *et al.* (1988) Molecular pathology of amyloid deposition in Alzheimer's disease, in *Etiology of Dementia of Alzheimer's type* (eds A.S. Henderson and J.H. Henderson), John Wiley, Chichester.

Bharucha, N.E., Schoenberg, B.S. and Kokmen, E. (1983) Dementia of Alzheimer's type (DAT): a case-control study of association with medical conditions and surgical procedures. *Neurology*, **33**, 85.

Bickel, H. and Cooper, B. (1989) Incidence of dementing illness among persons aged over 65 in an urban population, in *Epidemiology and The Prevention of Mental Disorders* (eds B. Cooper and T. Helgason), Routledge, London.

Birkett, D.P. (1972) The psychiatric differentiation of senility and arteriosclerosis. *Br. J. Psychiatry*, **120**, 321–5.

Bland, R.C., Newman, S.C. and Orn, H. (1988) Prevalence of psychiatric disorders in the elderly in Edmonton. *Acta Psychiatr. Scand.*, **77** (suppl. 338), 57–63.

Blessed, G., Tomlinson, B.E. and Roth, M. (1968) The association between quantitative measures of dementia and of senile change in the cerebral grey matter of elderly subjects. *Br. J. Psychiatry*, **114**, 797–811.

Blessed, G. and Wilson, I.D. (1982) The contemporary natural history of mental disorder in old age. *Br. J. Psychiatry*, **141**, 59–67.

Boller, F., Vrtunski, B., Mack, J.L. and Kim, Y. (1977) Neuropsychological correlates of hypertension. *Arch. Neurol.*, **34**, 701–5.

Boller, F., Lopez, O.L. and Moossy, J. (1989) Diagnosis of dementia: Clinicopathologic correlations. *Neurology*, **39**, 76–9.

Bollerup, T.R. (1975) Prevalence of mental illness among 70-year-olds domiciled in nine Copenhagen suburbs. *Acta Psychiatr. Scand.*, **51**, 327–39.

Bond, J. (1987) Psychiatric illness in later life. A study of prevalence in a Scottish population. *Int. J. Geriatr. Psychiatry*, **2**, 39–57.

Bondareff, W. (1983) Age and Alzheimer disease. *Lancet*, **i**, 1447.

Bradburn, N.M., Rips, L.J. and Shevell, S.K. (1987) Answering autobiographical questions: The impact of memory and inference on surveys. *Science*, **236**, 157–61.

Brayne, C. and Calloway, P. (1988) Normal ageing, impaired cognitive function, and senile dementia of the Alzheimer's type: A continuum? *Lancet*, **ii**, 1265–7.

Brayne, C. and Calloway, P. (1989) An epidemiological study of dementia in a rural population of elderly women. *Br. J. Psychiatry*, **155**, 214–19.

Breitner, J.C.S. and Folstein, M.F. (1984) Familial Alzheimer dementia: A prevalent disorder with specific clinical features. *Psychol. Med.*, **14**, 63–80.

Breitner, J.C.S., Folstein, M.F. and Murphy, E.A. (1986) Familial aggregation in Alzheimer dementia – 1: A model for the age-dependent expression of an autosomal dominant gene. *J. Psychiatr. Res.*, **20**, 31–43.

Bremer, J. (1951) A social psychiatric investigation of a small community in Northern Norway. *Acta Psychiatr. Neurologica Scand.*, (suppl. 62).

Brody, J.A. and Schneider, E.L. (1986) Diseases and disorders of aging: An hypothesis. *J. Chronic Dis.*, **39**, 871–6.

Broe, G.A. (1988) Alzheimer's disease and brain ageing, in *Proceedings of IV International Meeting of Alzheimer's Disease International* (ed. F. Jordan), Alzheimer's Disease and Related Disorders Society of Australia, Brisbane.

Broe, G.A., Akhtar, A.J., Andrews, G.R. *et al.* (1976) Neurological disorders in the elderly at home. *J. Neurol. Neurosurg. Psychiatry*, **39**, 362–6.

Broe, G.A., Henderson, A.S., McCusker, E. *et al.* (1990) A case-control study of Alzheimer's disease in Australia. Submitted to *Neurology*.

Brun, A. and Englund, E. (1986) A white matter disorder in dementia of the Alzheimer type: A pathoanatomical study. *Ann. Neurol.*, **19**, 253–62.

Bucht, G., Adolfsson, R. and Winblad, B. (1984) Dementia of the Alzheimer type and multi-infarct dementia: A clinical description and diagnostic problems. *J. Am. Geriatr. Soc.*, **32**, 491–8.

Burke, W.J., Miller, J.P., Rubin, E.H. *et al.* (1988) Reliability of the Washington University clinical dementia rating. *Arch. Neurol.*, **45**, 31–2.

Calne, D.B., Eisen, A., McGeer, E. and Spencer, P. (1986) Alzheimer's disease, Parkinson's disease, and motoneurone disease: Abiotropic interaction between ageing and environment? *Lancet*, **ii**, 1067–70.

Campbell, A.J., McCosh, L.M., Reinken, J. and Allan, B.C. (1983) Dementia in old age and the need for services. *Age Ageing*, **12**, 11–16.

Chandra, V., Bharucha, N.E. and Schoenberg, B.S. (1986a) Patterns of mortality from types of dementia in the United States, 1971 and 1973–1978. *Neurology*, **36**, 204–8.

Chandra, V., Bharucha, N.E. and Schoenberg, B. (1986b) Conditions associated with Alzheimer's disease at death: case-control study. *Neurology*, **36**, 209–11.

Chandra, V., Kokmen, E. and Schoenberg, B.S. (1987b) Head trauma with loss of consciousness as a risk factor for Alzheimer's disease using prospectively collected data. *Neurology*, **37** (suppl. 1), 152.

Chandra, V., Philipose, V., Bell, P.A. *et al.* (1987a) Case-control study of late onset 'probable Alzheimer's disease'. *Neurology*, **37**, 1295–300.

Chase, G.A., Folstein, M.F., Breitner, J.C.S. *et al.* (1983) The use of life tables and survival analysis in testing genetic hypotheses, with an application to Alzheimer's disease. *Am. J. Epidemiol.*, **117**, 590–7.

Chen, X.S. (1987) An epidemiologic investigation of mental disorders of the aged in an urban district of Beijing. *Chin. J. Neurol. Psychiatry*, **20**, 145–50 (in Chinese).

Christie, A.B. (1982) Changing patterns in mental illness in the elderly. *Br. J. Psychiatry*, **140**, 154–9.

Christie, A.B. and Train, J.D. (1984) Change in the pattern of care for the demented. *Br. J. Psychiatry*, **144**, 9–15.

Chui, H.C., Teng, E.L., Henderson, V.W. and Moy, A.C. (1985) Clinical subtypes of dementia of the Alzheimer type. *Neurology*, **35**, 1544–50.

Clark, I.A., Cowden, W.B. and Hunt, N.H. (1985) Free radical-induced pathology. *Med. Res. Rev.*, **5**, 297–332.

Clarke, M., Lowry, R. and Clarke, S. (1986) Cognitive impairment in the elderly – a community survey. *Age and Ageing*, **15**, 278–84.

Cohen, D., Eisdorfer, C. and Leverenz, J. (1982) Alzheimer's disease and maternal age. *J. Am. Geriatr. Soc.*, **30**, 656–9.

Constantinidis, J. (1978) Is Alzheimer's disease a major form of senile dementia? Clinical, anatomical, and genetic data, in *Alzheimer's Disease: Senile dementia and related disorders* (eds R. Katzman, R.D. Terry and K.L. Bick), Raven Press, New York.

Cooper, B. (1984) Home and away: The disposition of mentally ill old people in an urban population. *Soc. Psychiatry*, **19**, 187–96.

Copeland, J.R.M., Kelleher, M.J., Kellett, J.M. *et al.* (1976) A semi-structured clinical interview for the assessment of diagnosis and mental state in the elderly: The Geriatric Mental State Schedule. I. Development and reliability. *Psychol. Med.*, **6**, 439–49.

Copeland, J.R.M., Dewey, M.E. and Griffiths-Jones, H.M. (1986) Computerised psychiatric diagnostic system and case nomenclature for elderly persons. GMS and AGECAT. *Psychol. Med.*, **16**, 89–99.

Copeland, J.R.M., Gurland, B.J., Dewey, M.E. *et al.* (1987a) Is there more dementia, depression and neurosis in New York? A comparative study of the elderly in New York and London using the computer diagnosis AGECAT. *Br. J. Psychiatry*, **151**, 466–73.

Copeland, J.R.M., Dewey, M.E., Wood, N. *et al.* (1987b) Range of mental illness among the elderly in the community: Prevalence in Liverpool using the GMS-AGECAT package. *Br. J. Psychiatry*, **150**, 815–23.

Copeland, J.R.M., Dewey, M.E., Henderson, A.S. *et al.* (1988) The Geriatric Mental State (GMS) used in the community: replication studies of the computerized diagnosis AGECAT. *Psychol. Med.*, **18**, 219–23.

Coquoz, D. (1984) Epidemiology of senile dementia, in *Senile Dementia: Outlook for the future* (eds J. Wertheimer and M. Marois), Alan R. Liss, New York.

Coriat, A.M. and Gillard, R.D. (1986) Beware the cups that cheer. *Nature*, **321**, 570.

Corkin, S., Growdon, J.H. and Rasmussen, S.L. (1983) Parental age as a risk factor in Alzheimer's disease. *Ann. Neurol,,* **13**, 674–6.

Corsellis, J. (1978) Posttraumatic dementia, in *Alzheimer Disease: Senile dementia and related disorders* (eds R. Katzman, R.D. Terry and K.L. Bick), Raven Press, New York.

Creasey, H. and Rapoport, S.I. (1985) The aging human brain. *Ann. Neurol.,* **17**, 2–10.

Creasey, H., Jorm, A. Longley, W. *et al.* (1989) Monozygotic twins discordant for Alzheimer's disease. *Neurology,* **39**, 1474–6.

Cummings, J.L. and Benson, D.F. (1983) *Dementia: A clinical approach.* Butterworths, Boston.

Cummins, R.A., Walsh, R.N., Budtz-Olsen, O.E. *et al.* (1973) Environmentally-induced changes in the brains of elderly rats. *Nature,* **243**, 516–18.

D'Alessandro, R., Gallassi, R., Benassi, G. *et al.* (1988) Dementia in subjects over 65 years of age in the Republic of San Marino. *Br. J. Psychiatry,* **153**, 182–6.

Dalton, A.J., Crapper, D.R. and Schlotterer, G.R. (1974) Alzheimer's disease in Down's syndrome: Visual retention deficits. *Cortex,* **10**, 366–77.

Davies, L., Wolska, B., Hilbich, C. *et al.* (1988) A4 amyloid protein deposition and the diagnosis of Alzheimer's disease: Prevalence in aged brains determined by immunocytochemistry compared with conventional neuropathologic techniques. *Neurology,* **38**, 1688–93.

De Braekeleer, M., Froda, S., Gautrin, D. *et al.* (1988) Parental age and birth order in Alzheimer's disease: A case-control study in the Saguenay-Lac-St-Jean area (Quebec, Canada). *Can. J. Neurol. Sci.,* **15**, 139–41.

Delabar, J-M., Goldgaber, D., Lamour, Y. *et al.* (1987) β amyloid gene duplication in Alzheimer's disease and karyotypically normal Down syndrome. *Science,* **235**, 1390–2.

de Leon, M.J., La Regina, M.E., Ferris, S.H. *et al.* (1986) Reduced incidence of left-handedness in clinically diagnosed dementia of the Alzheimer type. *Neurobiol. Aging,* **7**, 161–4.

Dewey, M.E., Davidson, I.A. and Copeland, J.R.M. (1988) Risk factors for dementia: Evidence from the Liverpool study of continuing health in the community. *Int. J. Geriatr. Psychiatry,* **3**, 245–9.

Diesfeldt, H.F.A., van Houte, L.R. and Moerkens, R.M. (1986) Duration of survival in senile dementia. *Acta Psychiatr. Scand.,* **73**, 366–71.

Dilling, H. and Weyerer, S. (1984) Prevalence of mental disorders in the small-town – rural region of Traunstein (Upper Bavaria). *Acta Psychiatr. Scand.,* **69**, 60–79.

Dixon, B. (1988) Scientifically speaking. *Br. Med. J.,* **296**, 650.

Dormandy, T.L. (1988) In praise of peroxidation. *Lancet,* **ii**, 1126–8.

Drexler, E.D., Miller, A.E. and Keilson, M.J. (1984) Left-handedness in dementia. *Neurology*, **34**, 1622.

Duckworth, G.S., Kedward, H.B. and Bailey, W.F. (1979) Prognosis of mental illness in old age: a four year follow-up study. *Can. J. Psychiatr.*, **24**, 674–82.

Dyken, M.L., Wolf, P.A., Barnett, H.J.M. *et al.* (1984) Risk factors in stroke. A statement for physicians by the Subcommittee on Risk Factors and Stroke of the Stroke Council. *Stroke*, **15**, 1105–11.

Eaton, W.W., Kramer, M., Anthony, J.C. *et al.* (1989) The incidence of specific DIS/DSM-III mental disorders: data from the NIMH Epidemiologic Catchment Area Program. *Acta Psychiatr. Scand.*, **79**, 163–78.

Ebrahim, S. (1989) Aluminium and Alzheimer's disease. *Lancet*, **i**, 267.

Edwardson, J.A., Klinowski, J., Oakley, A.E. *et al.* (1986) Aluminosilicates and the aging brain: Implications for the pathogenesis of Alzheimer's disease, in *1986 Silicon Biochemistry*, (Ciba Foundation Symposium 121), John Wiley, Chichester.

Engedal, K., Gilje, K. and Laake, K. (1988) Prevalence of dementia in a Norwegian sample aged 75 years and over and living at home. *Comprehensive Gerontology Series A*, **2**, 102–6.

English, D. and Cohen, D. (1985) A case-control study of maternal age in Alzheimer's disease. *J. Am. Geriatr. Soc.*, **33**, 167–9.

Erkinjuntti, T., Sulkava, R. and Tilvis, R. (1985) HDL-cholesterol in dementia. *Lancet*, **ii**, 43.

Erkinjuntti, T., Partinen, M., Sulkava, R. *et al.* (1987a) Snoring and dementia. *Age Ageing*, **16**, 305–10.

Erkinjuntti, T., Sulkava, R., Kovanen, J. and Palo, J. (1987b) Suspected dementia: evaluation of 323 consecutive referrals. *Acta Neurol. Scand.*, **76**, 359–64.

Erkinjuntti, T., Partinen, M., Sulkava, R. *et al.* (1987c) Sleep apnea in multiinfarct dementia and Alzheimer's disease. *Sleep*, **10**, 419–25.

Erkinjuntti, T., Haltia, M., Palo, J. *et al.* (1988) Accuracy of the clinical diagnosis of vascular dementia: a prospective clinical and post-mortem neuropathological study. *J. Neurol. Neurosurg. Psychiatry*, **51**, 1037–44.

Errebo-Knudsen, E.O. and Olsen, F. (1986) Organic solvents and presenile dementia (the painters' syndrome). A critical review of the Danish literature. *Sci. Total Environ.*, **48**, 45–67.

Escobar, J.I., Burnam, A., Karno, M. *et al.* (1986) Use of the Mini-Mental State Examination (MMSE) in a community population of mixed ethnicity: Cultural and linguistic artifacts. *J. Nerv. Ment. Dis.*, **174**, 607–14.

Esiri, M. (1982) Viruses and Alzheimer's disease. *J. Neurol. Neurosurg. Psychiatry*, **45**, 759.

Esiri, M.M. and Wilcock, G.K. (1984) The olfactory bulbs in Alzheimer's disease. *J. Neurol. Neurosurg. Psychiatry*, **47**, 56–60.

Essen-Möller, E., Larsson, H., Uddenberg, C.E. and White, G. (1956) Individual traits and morbidity in a Swedish rural population. *Acta Psychiatr. Scand.* (suppl. 100), 5–160.

Evans, D.A., Funkenstein, H.H., Albert, M.S. *et al.* (1990) Prevalence of Alzheimer's disease in a community population of older persons: Higher than previously reported. *J. Am. Med. Assoc.*, **262**, 2551–6.

Fairweather-Tait, S.J., Moore, G.R. and Fatemi, S.E.J. (1987) Low levels of aluminium in tea. *Nature*, **330**, 213.

Ferini-Strambi, L., Smirme, S., Truci, G. and Franceschi, M. (1987) Alzheimer's disease: clinical and epidemiological aspects in patients with early onset of the disease. *Clin. Neurol. Neurosurg.*, **89** (suppl. 2), 10–11.

Fillenbaum, G.G., Hughes, D.C., Heyman, A. *et al.* (1988) Relationship of health and demographic characteristics to Mini-Mental State Examination score among community residents. *Psychol. Med.*, **18**, 719–26.

Filley, C.M., Brownell, H.H. and Albert, M.L. (1985) Education provides no protection against Alzheimer's disease. *Neurology*, **35**, 1781–4.

Filley, C.M., Kelly, J. and Heaton, R.K. (1986) Neuropsychologic features of early- and late-onset Alzheimer's disease. *Arch. Neurol.*, **43**, 574–6.

Fisher, C.M. (1968) Dementia in cerebral vascular disease, in *Cerebral vascular disease* (eds J.F. Toole, R.G. Siekert and J.P. Whisnant), Grune & Stratton, New York.

Fisher, M.A. and Zeaman, D. (1970) Growth and decline of retardate intelligence, in *International review of research in mental retardation* (ed. N.R. Ellis), (Vol. 4), Academic Press, New York.

Fitch, N., Becker, R. and Heller, A. (1988) The inheritance of Alzheimer's disease: a new interpretation. *Ann. Neurol.*, **23**, 14–19.

Flaten, T.P. (1987) Geographical associations between aluminium in drinking water and registered death rates with dementia (including Alzheimer's disease) in Norway, in *Proceedings from the Second International Symposium on Geochemistry and Health*, London.

Flaten, T.P. (1989) Mortality from dementia in Norway, 1969–85. *J. Epidemiol. Commun. Health*, **43**, 285–9.

Flynn, J.R. (1984) The mean IQ of Americans: Massive gains 1932 to 1978. *Psychol. Bull.*, **95**, 29–51.

Flynn, J.R. (1987) Massive IQ gains in 14 nations: What IQ tests really measure. *Psychol. Bull.*, **101**, 171–91.

Folstein, M.F., Folstein, S.E. and McHugh, P.R. (1975) 'Mini-Mental State': A practical method for grading the cognitive state of patients for the clinician. *J. Psychiatr. Res.*, **12**, 189–98.

Folstein, M.F. and McHugh, P.R. (1978) Dementia syndrome of depression, in *Alzheimer's Disease: Senile dementia and related disorders* (eds

R. Katzman, R.D. Terry and K.L. Bick). (*Aging*, Vol. 7), Raven Press, New York.

Folstein, M.F. and Breitner, J.C. (1981) Language disorder predicts familial Alzheimer's disease. *Johns Hopkins Med. J.*, **149**, 145–7.

Folstein, M.F., Anthony, J.C., Parhad, I. *et al.* (1985) The meaning of cognitive impairment in the elderly. *J. Am. Geriatr. Soc.*, **33**, 228–35.

Foncin, J.F. (1987) Alzheimer's disease and aluminium. *Nature*, **326**, 136.

Franceschi, M., Tancredi, D., Smirne, S. *et al.* (1982) Cognitive processes in hypertension. *Hypertension*, **4**, 226–9.

Freemon, F.R. (1976) Evaluation of patients with progressive intellectual deterioration. *Arch. Neurol.*, **33**, 658–9.

French, L.R., Schuman, L.M., Mortimer, J.A. *et al.* (1985) A case-control study of dementia of the Alzheimer type. *Am. J. Epidemiol.*, **121**, 414–21.

French, L.R., Schuman, L.M., Mortimer, J.A. and Hutton, J.T. (1986) The authors reply. *Am. J. Epidemiol.*, **123**, 753–4.

Gaillard, M. (1984) Epidemiological elements in presenile Alzheimer's disease, in *Senile Dementia: Outlook for the Future* (eds J. Wertheimer and M. Marois). Alan R. Liss, New York, pp. 411–25.

Gajdusek, D.C. (1977) Unconventional viruses and the origin and disappearance of kuru. *Science*, **197**, 943–60.

Garraway, W.M., Whisnant, J.P., Furlan, A.J. *et al.* (1979) The declining incidence of stroke. *New Engl. J. Med.*, **300**, 449–52.

Gavrilova, S. (1984) Demonstrability of mental disorders in late middle and old age. *Zh. Nevropatol. Psikhiatr.*, **84**, 911–18 (in Russian).

Gavrilova, S.I., Sudareva, L.O., and Kalyn, Y.B. (1987) Epidemiology of dementias in the middle-aged and elderly. *Zh. Nevropatol. Psikhiatr.*, **87**, 1345–52 (in Russian).

Ghidoni, E., Chiessi, G., Dalbari, A. *et al.* (1987) Fingerprint patterns and genetic risk factors in Alzheimer's disease. *Neuroscience*, **22** (suppl.) S439.

Gibberd, F.B. and Simmonds, J.P. (1980) Neurological disease in ex-Far-East prisoners of war. *Lancet*, **ii**, 135–7.

Gilmore, A.J.J. (1974) Community services and mental health, in *Geriatric medicine* (eds W.F. Anderson and T.G. Judge), Academic Press, London.

Go, R.C.P., Todorov, A.B., Elston, R.C. and Constantinidis, J. (1978) The malignancy of dementias. *Ann. Neurol.*, **3**, 559–61.

Goate, A.M., Haynes, A.R., Owen, M.J. *et al.* (1989) Predisposing locus for Alzheimer's disease on chromosome 21. *Lancet*, **i**, 352–5.

Golden, R.R., Teresi, J.A. and Gurland, B.J. (1983) Detection of dementia and depression cases with the Comprehensive Assessment and Referral Evaluation interview schedule. *Int. J. Aging Hum. Dev.*, **16**, 241–54.

Goldgaber, D., Lerman, M.I., McBride, O.W. *et al.* (1987) Characterization and chromosomal localization of a cDNA encoding brain amyloid of Alzheimer's disease. *Science*, **235**, 877–80.

Goodman, L. (1953) Alzheimer's disease: A clinico-pathologic analysis of twenty-three cases with a theory of pathogenesis. *J. Nerv. Ment. Dis.*, **117**, 97–130.

Goudsmit, J., Morrow, C.H., Asher, D.M. *et al.* (1980) Evidence for and against the transmissibility of Alzheimer disease. *Neurology*, **30**, 945–50.

Graves, A.B., White, E., Koepsell, T. and Reifler, B. (1987) A case-control study of Alzheimer's disease. *Am. J. Epidemiol.*, **126**, 754.

Greenhouse, A.H. (1982) Heavy metals and the nervous system. *Clin. Neuropharmacol.*, **5**, 45–92.

Greenland, S. (1987) Quantitative methods in the review of epidemiologic literature. *Epidemiol. Rev.*, **9**, 1–30.

Griffiths, R.A., Good, W.R., Watson, N.P. *et al.* (1987) Depression, dementia and disability in the elderly. *Br. J. Psychiatry*, **150**, 482–93.

Gruenberg, E.M. (1961) A mental health survey of older persons, in *Comparative epidemiology of mental disorders* (eds P.H. Hoch and J. Zubin), Grune & Stratton, New York.

Gruenberg, E.M. (1977) The failures of success. *Milbank Memorial Fund Quarterly*, **55**, 3–24.

Gruer, R. (1975) *Needs of the elderly in the Scottish borders*, Scottish Health Services Studies No. 33, Scottish Home and Health Department, Edinburgh.

Gunner-Svensson, F. and Jensen, K. (1976) Frequency of mental disorders in old age. Examples of comparability of epidemiological investigations in relation to utility in planning. *Acta Psychiatr. Scand.*, **53**, 283–97.

Gurland, B.J. (1981) The borderlands of dementia: The influence of sociocultural characteristics on rates of dementia occurring in the senium, in *Clinical Aspects of Alzheimer's Disease and Senile Dementia* (eds N.E. Miller and G.D. Cohen), (*Aging*, Vol. 15), Raven Press, New York.

Gurland, B., Kuriansky, J., Sharpe, L. *et al.* (1977a) The Comprehensive Assessment and Referral Evaluation (CARE) – rationale, development and reliability. *Int. J. Aging Hum. Dev.*, **8**, 9–42.

Gurland, B., Copeland, J., Sharpe, L. *et al.* (1977b) Assessment of the older person in the community. *Int. J. Aging Hum. Dev.*, **8**, 1–8.

Gurland, B.J., Dean, L.L., Copeland, J. *et al.* (1982) Criteria for the diagnosis of dementia in the community elderly. *Gerontologist*, **22**, 180–6.

Gurland, B., Copeland, J., Kuriansky, J. *et al.* (1983) *The Mind and Mood of Aging*, Croom Helm, London.

Gurland, B., Golden, R.R., Teresi, J.A. and Challop, J. (1984) The SHORT-CARE: An efficient instrument for the assessment of depression, dementia and disability. *J. Gerontol.*, **39**, 166–9.

Gustafson, L. and Nilsson, L. (1982) Differential diagnosis of presenile dementia on clinical grounds. *Acta Psychiatr. Scand.*, **65**, 194–209.

Habbema, J.D.F. and Dippel, D.W.J. (1986) Survivors-only bias in estimating survival in Alzheimer's disease and vascular dementias. *Neurology*, **36**, 1009.

Haberman, S., Capildeo, R. and Rose, F.C. (1981) Sex differences in the incidence of cerebrovascular disease. *J. Epidemiol. Commun. Health*, **35**, 45–50.

Hachinski, V.C., Lassen, N.A. and Marshall, J. (1974) Multi-infarct dementia: a cause of mental deterioration in the elderly. *Lancet*, **ii**, 207–10.

Hachinski, V.C. Iliff, L.D., Zilhka, E. *et al.* (1975) Cerebral blood flow in dementia. *Arch. Neurol.*, **32**, 632–7.

Hagnell, O., Lanke, J. and Rorsman, B. (1981) Increasing prevalence and decreasing incidence of age psychoses. A longitudinal epidemiological investigation of a Swedish population: the Lundby study, in *Epidemiology and Prevention of Mental Illness in Old Age* (eds G. Magnussen, J. Nielsen and J. Buch), Nordisk Samråd for Ældreaktivitet, Hellerup.

Hagnell, O., Lanke, J., Rorsman, B. *et al.* (1983) Current trends in the incidence of senile and multi-infarct dementia. *Arch. Psychiatr. Neurol. Sci.*, **233**, 423–38.

Halliwell, B. and Gutteridge, J.M.C. (1985) Oxygen radicals and the nervous system. *Trends Neurol. Sci.*, **8**, 22–6.

Halliwell, B. and Gutteridge, J.M.C. (1986) Aluminosilicates and Alzheimer's disease. *Lancet*, **i**, 682.

Harman, D. (1985) Role of free radicals in aging and disease, in *Relations between Normal Aging and Disease* (ed. H.A. Johnson), Raven Press, New York.

Hasegawa, K. (1983) The clinical assessment of dementia in the aged: A dementia screening scale for psychogeriatric patients, in *Aging in the Eighties and Beyond* (eds M. Bergener, U. Lehr, E. Lang and R. Schmitz-Scherzer), Springer, New York.

Hasegawa, K., Iwai, H., Amamoto, H. *et al.* (1983) The epidemiological study on the psychogeriatric disorders, in *N. Shinfuku Memorial Volume for Retirement* (in Japanese).

Hasegawa, K., Homma, A. and Imai, Y. (1986) An epidemiological study of age-related dementia in the community. *Int. J. Geriatr. Psychiatry*, **1**, 45–55.

Helgason, L. (1977) Psychiatric services and mental illness in Iceland. *Acta Psychiatr. Scand.* (suppl. 268).

Helgason, T. (1973) Epidemiology of mental disorders in Iceland: A geriatric follow-up (preliminary report). *Excerpta Medica International Congress Series*, **274**, 350–7.

Henderson, A.S. (1983) The coming epidemic of dementia. *Aust. N. Z. J. Psychiatry*, **17**, 117–27.

Henderson, A.S. (1988) The risk factors for Alzheimer's disease: A review and a hypothesis. *Acta Psychiatr. Scand.*, **78**, 257–75.

Henderson, A.S. and Huppert, F.A. (1984) The problem of mild dementia. *Psychol. Med.*, **14**, 5–11.

Henderson, A.S. and Jorm, A.F. (1987) Is case-ascertainment of Alzheimer's disease in field surveys practicable? *Psychol. Med.*, **17**, 549–55.

Henderson, A.S. and Kay, D.W.K. (1984) The epidemiology of mental disorders in the aged, in *Handbook of Studies on Psychiatry and Old Age* (eds D.W.K. Kay and G.D. Burrows), Elsevier, Amsterdam.

Henderson, A.S., Duncan-Jones, P. and Finlay-Jones, R.A. (1983) The reliability of the Geriatric Mental State Examination. *Acta Psychiatr. Scand.*, **67**, 281–9.

Hendrie, H.C., Hall, K.S., Brittain, H.M. *et al.* (1988) The CAMDEX: A standardized instrument for the diagnosis of mental disorder in the elderly: A replication with a US sample. *J. Am. Geriatr. Soc.*, **36**, 402–8.

Heston, L.L. (1981) Genetic studies of dementia: with emphasis on Parkinson's disease and Alzheimer's neuropathology, in *The Epidemiology of Dementia* (eds J.A. Mortimer and L.M. Schuman), Oxford University Press, New York.

Heston, L.L. and White, J.A. (1983) *Dementia: A Practical Guide to Alzheimer's Disease and Related Illnesses*, W.H. Freeman, New York.

Hewitt, K.E., Carter, G. and Jancar, J. (1985) Ageing in Down's syndrome. *Br. J. Psychiatry*, **147**, 58–62.

Heyman, A., Wilkinson, W.E., Hurwitz, B.J. *et al.* (1983) Alzheimer's disease: Genetic aspects and associated clinical disorders. *Ann. Neurol.*, **14**, 507–15.

Heyman, A., Wilkinson, W.E., Stafford, J.A. *et al.* (1984) Alzheimer's disease: A study of epidemiological aspects. *Ann. Neurol.*. **15**. 335–41.

Heyman, A., Wilkinson, W.E., Hurwitz, B.J. *et al.* (1987) Early-onset Alzheimer's disease: Clinical predictors of institutionalization and death. *Neurology*, **37**, 980–4.

Hoch, C.C., Reynolds, C.F., Kupfer, D.J. *et al.* (1986) Sleep-disordered breathing in normal and pathologic aging. *J. Clin. Psychiatry*, **47**, 499–503.

Hodkinson, H.M. (1972) Evaluation of a mental test score for assessment of mental impairment in the elderly. *Age Ageing*, **1**, 233–8.

Hofman, A. (1987) Prevalence, incidence, prognosis and risk factors of dementia. *Rev. Epidemiol. Santé Publique*, **35**, 287–91.

Hofman, A., Schulte, W., Tanja, T.A. *et al.* (1989a) History of dementia in first-degree relatives and the risk of Alzheimer's disease. Unpublished manuscript, Erasmus University Medical School, Rotterdam.

Hofman, A., van Duijn, C.M., Schulte, W. *et al.* (1989b) Is parental age related to the risk of Alzheimer's disease? Unpublished manuscript, Erasmus University Medical School, Rotterdam.

Holzer, C.E., Tischler, G.L., Leaf, P.J. and Myers, J.K. (1984) An epidemiologic assessment of cognitive impairment in a community population, in *Research in Community and Mental Health* (Vol. 4), JAI Press, Greenwich, Connecticut.

Homer, A.C., Honavar, M., Lantos, P.L. *et al.* (1988) Diagnosing dementia: Do we get it right? *Br. Med. J.*, **297**, 896–6.

Huff, F.J., Auerbach, J., Chakravarti, A. and Boller, F. (1988) Risk of dementia in relatives of patients with Alzheimer's disease. *Neurology*, **38**, 786–90.

Hughes, C.P., Berg, L., Danziger, W.L. *et al.* (1982) A new clinical scale for the staging of dementia. *Br. J. Psychiatry*, **140**, 566–72.

Huppert, F.A. (1988) Age-related changes in memory: Learning and remembering new information, in *Handbook of Neuropsychology*, (eds F. Boller and J. Grafman), Elsevier, Amsterdam.

Hutton, J.T. (1981) Results of clinical assessment for the dementia syndrome: Implications for epidemiologic studies, in *The Epidemiology of Dementia* (eds J.A. Mortimer and L.M. Schuman), Oxford University Press, New York.

Ichinowatari, N., Tatsunuma, T. and Makiya, H. (1987) Epidemiological study of old age mental disorders in the two rural areas of Japan. *Jpn J. Psychiatr. Neurol.*, **41**, 629–36.

Iivanainen, M. (1975) Statistical correlations of diffuse cerebral atrophy, with special reference to diagnostic and aetiological clues. *Acta Neurol. Scand.*, **51**, 365–79.

Ineichen, B. (1987) Measuring the rising tide: How many dementia cases will there be by 2001? *Br. J. Psychiatry*, **150**, 193–200.

Israel, L., Kozarevic, D. and Sartorius, N. (1984) *Source Book of Geriatric Assessment*, Karger, Basle.

Jackson, J.A., Riordan, H.D. and Poling, C.M. (1989) Aluminium from a coffee pot. *Lancet*, **i**, 781–2.

Jacobs, J.W., Bernhard, M.R., Delgardo, A. and Strain, J.J. (1977) Screening for organic mental syndromes in the medically ill. *Ann. Intern. Med.*, **86**, 40–6.

Jagger, C., Clarke, M. and Cook, A.J. (1989) Mental and physical health of elderly people: Five-year follow-up of a total population. *Age and Ageing*, **18**, 77–82.

Jarvik, L.F. and Matsuyama, S.S. (1983) Parental stroke: Risk factor for multi-infarct dementia? *Lancet*, **ii**, 1025.

Jellinger, K. (1976) Neuropathological aspects of dementias resulting from abnormal blood and cerebrospinal fluid dynamics. *Acta Neurol. Belg.*, **76**, 83–102.

Jensen, A.R. (1980) *Bias in Mental Testing*, Methuen, London.

Jensen, G.D. and Polloi, A.H. (1988) The very old of Palau: Health and mental state. *Age Ageing*, **17**, 220–6.

Jensen, K. (1963) Psychiatric problems in four Danish old age homes. *Acta Psychiatr. Scand. (suppl. 169)*, 411–19.

Jensen, T.S., Genefke, I.K., Hyldebrandt, N. *et al.* (1982) Cerebral atrophy in young torture victims. *New Engl. J. Med.* **307**, 1341.

Jessen, G. and Svennild, I. (1986) Undersøgelse vedrørende øget forekomst af præsenil demens hos lastoptagere af industrifisk på Esbjerg havn. *Ugeskr. Læg.*, **148**, 2581–4.

Joachim, C.L., Morris, J.H. and Selkoe, D.J. (1988) Clinically diagnosed Alzheimer's disease: Autopsy results in 150 cases. *Ann. of Neurol.*, **24**, 50–6.

Jones, G.M.M., Reith, M., Philpot, M.P. and Sahakian, B.J. (1987) Smoking and dementia of Alzheimer type. *J. Neurol. Neurosurg. Psychiatry*, **50**, 1383.

Jorm, A.F. (1985) Subtypes of Alzheimer's dementia: A conceptual analysis and critical review. *Psychol. Med.*, **15**, 543–53.

Jorm, A.F. (1989) Some pitfalls in data analysis, in *Alzheimer's Disease* (eds R.J. Wurtman, S. Corkin, J.H. Growdon and E. Ritter-Walker), Proceedings of the Fifth Meeting of the International Study Group on the Pharmacology of Memory Disorders Associated with Aging, Zurich.

Jorm, A.F. and Henderson, A.S. (1985) Possible improvements to the diagnostic criteria for dementia in DSM-III. *Br. J. Psychiatry*, **147**, 394–9.

Jorm, A.F. and Korten, A.E. (1988) A method for calculating projected increases in the number of dementia sufferers – with application to Australia and New Zealand. *Aust. N. Z. J. Psychiatry*, **22**, 183–9.

Jorm, A.F., Korten, A.E. and Henderson, A.S. (1987) The prevalence of dementia: a quantitative integration of the literature. *Acta Psychiatr. Scand.*, **76**, 465–79.

Jorm, A.F., Scott, R., Henderson, A.S. and Kay, D.W.K. (1988a) Educational level differences on the Mini-Mental State: The role of test bias. *Psychol. Med.*, **18**, 727–31.

Jorm, A.F., Korten, A.E. and Jacomb, P.A. (1988b) Projected increases in the number of dementia cases for 29 developed countries: Application of a new method for making projections. *Acta Psychiatr. Scand.*, **78**, 493–500.

Jorm, A.F., Henderson, A.S. and Jacomb, P.A. (1989) Regional differences in mortality from dementia in Australia: An analysis of death certificate data. *Acta Psychiatr. Scand.*, **79**, 179–85.

Jouan-Flahault, C., Seroussi, M.C. and Colvez, A. (1989) Absence de liaison entre démence sénile et âge parental. *Rev. Epidémiol. Santé Publique*, **37**, 73–5.

Kagan, A., Popper, J., Rhoads, G.G. *et al.* (1976) Epidemiologic studies of coronary heart disease and stroke in Japanese men living in Japan, Hawaii, and California: Prevalence of stroke, in *Cerebrovascular Diseases* (ed. P. Scheinberg), Raven Press, New York.

Kahn, R.L., Goldfarb, A.I., Pollack, M. and Peck, A. (1960) Brief objective measures for the determination of mental status in the aged. *Am. J. Psychiatry*, **117**, 326–8.

Kahn, R.L., Pollack, M. and Goldfarb, A.I. (1961) Factors related to individual differences in mental status of institutionalized aged, in *Psychopathology of Aging* (eds P.H. Hoch and J. Zubin), Grune & Stratton, New York.

Kaneko, (1975) Care in Japan, in *Modern Perspectives in the Psychiatry of Old Age* (ed. J.G. Howells), Brunner-Mazel, New York.

Karasawa, A., Kawashima, K. and Kasahara, H. (1982) Epidemiological study of the senile in Tokyo metropolitan area. *Proceedings of World Psychiatric Association Regional Symposium*, 285–9.

Kato, M. (1969) Psychiatric epidemiological surveys in Japan: The problem of case finding, in *Mental Health Research in Asia and the Pacific* (eds W. Caudell and T. Lin). East-West Center Press, Honolulu.

Katzman, R. (1976) The prevalence and malignancy of Alzheimer's disease. A major killer. *Arch. Neurol.*, **33**, 217–18.

Katzman, R., Terry, R., De Teresa, R. *et al.* (1988) Clinical, pathological, and neurochemical changes in dementia: A subgroup with preserved mental status and numerous neocortical plaques. *Ann. Neurol.*, **23**, 138–44.

Katzman, R., Aronson, M., Fuld, P. *et al.* (1989) Development of dementing illnesses in an 80-year-old volunteer cohort. *Ann. Neurol.*, **25**, 317–24.

Kay, D.W.K. (1962) Outcome and cause of death in mental disorders of old age: A long-term follow-up of functional and organic psychoses. *Acta Psychiatr. Scand.*, **38**, 249–76.

Kay, D.W.K., Beamish, P. and Roth, M. (1964a) Old age mental disorders in Newcastle upon Tyne, Part I. A study of prevalence. *Br. J. Psychiatry*, **110**, 146–58.

Kay, D.W.K., Beamish, P. and Roth, M. (1964b) Old age mental disorders in Newcastle upon Tyne. Part II. A study of possible social and medical causes. *Br. J. Psychiatry*, **110**, 668–82.

Kay, D.W.K. and Bergmann, K. (1980) Epidemiology of mental disorders among the aged in the community, in *Handbook of Mental Health and Aging* (eds J.E. Birren and R.B. Sloane), Prentice-Hall, Englewood Cliffs.

Kay, D.W.K., Bergmann, K., Foster, E.M. *et al.* (1970) Mental illness and hospital usage in the elderly: a random sample followed up. *Comprehensive Psychiatry*, **11**, 26–35.

Kay, D.W.K., Henderson, A.S., Scott, R. *et al.* (1985) Dementia and depression among the elderly living in the Hobart community: The effect of the diagnostic criteria on the prevalence rates. *Psychol. Med.*, **15**, 771–88.

Kellett, J.M. (1988) Aspirin and cyclandelate in multi infarct dementia, in *Proceedings of IV International Meeting of Alzheimer's Disease International* (ed. F. Jordan), Alzheimer's Disease and Related Disorders Society of Australia, Brisbane.

Khachaturian, Z.S. (1985) Diagnosis of Alzheimer's disease. *Arch. Neurol.*, **42**, 1097–105.

Kidd, C. (1962) Old people in mental hospitals: A study in diagnostic composition and outcome. *Ir. J. Med. Sci.*, **6**, 72–8.

Kidson, M.A. (1967) Psychiatric disorders in the Walbiri, Central Australia. *Aust. N. Z. J. Psychiatry*, **1**, 14–22.

Kittner, S.J., White, L.R., Farmer, M.E. *et al.* (1986) Methodological issues in screening for dementia: The problem of education adjustment. *J. Chronic Dis.*, **39**, 163–70.

Klatzo, I., Wisniewski, H. and Streicher, E. (1965) Experimental production of neurofibrillary degeneration. *J. Neuropathol. Exp. Neurol.*, **24**, 187–99.

Knesevich, J.W., LaBarge, E., Martin, R.L. *et al.* (1982) Birth order and maternal age effect in dementia of the Alzheimer type. *Psychiatr. Res.*, **7**, 345–50.

Knesevich, J.W., Toro, F.R., Morris, J.C. and LaBarge, E. (1985) Aphasia, family history, and the longitudinal course of senile dementia of the Alzheimer type. *Psychiatr. Res.*, **14**, 255–63.

Kokmen, E., Offord, K.P. and Okazaki, H. (1987) A clinical and autopsy study of dementia in Olmsted Country, Minnesota, 1980–1981. *Neurology*, **37**, 426–30.

Kokmen, E., Chandra, V. and Schoenberg, B.S. (1988) Trends in incidence of dementing illness in Rochester, Minnesota, in three quinquennial periods, 1960–1974. *Neurology*, **38**, 975–80.

Kokmen, E., Beard, M., Offord, K.P. and Kurland, L.T. (1989) Prevalence of medically diagnosed dementia in a defined United States population: Rochester, Minnesota, January 1, 1975. *Neurology*, **39**, 773–6.

Koning, J.H. (1981) Aluminum pots as a source of dietary aluminum. *New Engl. J. Med.*, **304**, 172–3.

Koss, E., Weiffenbach, J.M., Haxby, J.V. and Friedland, R.P. (1988) Olfactory detection and identification performance are dissociated in early Alzheimer's disease. *Neurology*, **38**, 1228–32.

Kramer, M. (1983) The increasing prevalence of mental disorder: A pandemic threat. *Psychiatr. Q.*, **55**, 115–43.

Kramer, M., German, P.S., Anthony, J.C. *et al.* (1985) Patterns of mental disorders among the elderly residents of eastern Baltimore. *J. Am. Geriatr. Soc.*, **33**, 236–45.

Kuang, P.G. and Zhao, Z.P. (1984) A survey of senile disturbances in Wuhen city in 1981. *Chin. J. Epidemiol.*, **5**, 95–9 (in Chinese).

Ladurner, G., Iliff, L.D. and Lechner, H. (1982) Clinical factors associated with dementia in ischaemic stroke. *J. Neurol. Neurosurg. Psychiatry*, **45**, 97–101.

Larson, E.B., Reifler, B.V., Sumi, S.M. *et al.* (1985) Diagnostic evaluation of 200 elderly outpatients with suspected dementia. *J. Gerontol.*, **40**, 536–43.

Larsson, T., Sjögren, T. and Jacobson, G. (1963) Senile dementia: A clinical, sociomedical and genetic study. *Acta Psychiatr. Scand.*, (suppl. 167), 1–259.

La Rue, A. and Jarvik, L.F. (1987) Cognitive function and prediction of dementia in old age. *Int. J. Aging Hum. Dev.*, **25**, 79–89.

Lehtonen, A. and Luutonen, S. (1986) High-density lipoprotein cholesterol levels of very old people in the diagnosis of dementia. *Age Ageing*, **15**, 267–70.

Leighton, D.C., Harding, J.S., Macklin *et al.* (1963) *The Character of Danger*, Basic Books, New York.

Levick, S.E. (1980) Dementia from aluminum pots? *New Engl. J. Med.*, **303**, 164.

Lewin, W., Marshall, T.F.D.C. and Roberts, A.H. (1979) Long-term outcome after severe head injury. *Br. Med. J.*, **2**, 1533–8.

Li, G., Shen, Y.C., Chen, C.H. *et al.* (1989) An epidemiological survey of age-related dementia in an urban area of Beijing. *Acta Psychiatr. Scand.*, **79**, 557–63.

Lin, T. (1953) A study of the incidence of mental disorder in Chinese and other cultures. *Psychiatry*, **16**, 313–36.

Lin, T., Rin, H., Yeh, E-K. *et al.* (1969) Mental disorders in Taiwan, fifteen years later: A preliminary report, in *Mental health Research in Asia and the Pacific* (eds W. Caudell and T. Lin), East–West Center Press, Honolulu.

Lindesay, J. (1989) Aluminium and Alzheimer's disease. *Lancet*, **i**, 268.

Lione, A., Allen, P.V. and Smith, J.C. (1984) Aluminium coffee percolators as a source of dietary aluminium. *Food and Chemical Toxicology*, **22**, 265–8.

Lippi, A., Rocca, W.A., Bonaiuto, S. *et al.* (1989) Prevalence of Alzheimer's disease (AD) and other dementing disorders: A door-to-door survey in Appignano, Macerata Province, Italy. *Neurology*, **39** (suppl. 1), 180.

Liston, E.H. and La Rue, A. (1983) Clinical differentiation of primary degenerative and multi-infarct dementia: A critical review of the evidence. Part II: Pathological studies. *Biol. Psychiatry*, **18**, 1467–84.

Liston, E.H. and La Rue, A. (1986) DSM-III diagnosis of multi-infarct dementia. *Compr. Psychiatry*, 27, 54–9.

Løchen, E.A. (1968) Psychometric patterns, in *Norwegian Concentration Camp Survivors* (ed. A. Strøm), Humanities Press, New York.

Loesch, D. (1981) Dermatoglyphic studies in the parents of trisomy 21 children. *Human Heredity*, **31**, 201–7.

Loring, D.W. and Largen, J.W. (1985) Neuropsychological patterns of presenile and senile dementia of the Alzheimer type. *Neuropsychologia*, **23**, 351–7.

Louis, T.A., Fineberg, H.V. and Mosteller, F. (1985) Findings for public health from meta-analyses. *Annu. Rev. Pub. Health*, **6**, 1–20.

Luxenberg, J.S., Plato, C.C., Fox, K.M. *et al.* (1988) Digital and palmar dermatoglyphics in dementia of the Alzheimer type. *Am. J. Med. Genet.*, **30**, 733–40.

Lycke, E., Norrby, R. and Roos, B-E. (1974) A serological study on mentally ill patients: With particular reference to the prevalence of herpes virus infections. *Br. J. Psychiatry*, **124**, 273–9.

McDermott, J.R. and Smith, A.I. (1978) Brain aluminium concentration in dialysis encephalopathy. *Lancet*, **i**, 901.

McHugh, P.R. and Folstein, M.F. (1979) Psychopathology of dementia: Implications for neuropathology, in *Congenital and Acquired Cognitive Disorders* (ed. R. Katzman), Raven Press, New York.

McKhann, G., Drachman, D., Folstein, M. *et al.* (1984) Clinical diagnosis of Alzheimer's disease: Report of the NINCDS–ADRDA Work Group under the auspices of Department of Health and Human Services Task Force on Alzheimer's Disease. *Neurology*, **34**, 939–44.

McLaughlin, A.I.G., Kazantzis, G., King, E. *et al.* (1962) Pulmonary fibrosis and encephalopathy associated with the inhalation of aluminium dust. *Br. J. Ind. Med.*, **19**, 253–63.

McPherson, F.M., Gamsu, C.V., Kiemle, G. *et al.* (1985) The concurrent validity of the survey version of the Clifton Assessment Procedures for the Elderly (CAPE). *Br. J. Psychiatry*, **24**, 83–91.

Magnusson, H. and Helgason, T. (1981) Epidemiology of mental disorders in the aged in Iceland, in *Epidemiology and Prevention of Mental Illness in Old Age* (eds G. Magnussen, J. Nielsen and J. Buch), Nordisk Samråd for Eldreaktivitet, Hellerup, Denmark.

Makiya, H. (1978) An epidemiological investigation on the psychiatric disorders of the old age in Sashiki-village in Okinawa-prefecture. *Keio J. Med.*, **55**, 503–12 (in Japanese).

Malamud, N. (1972) Neuropathology of organic brain syndromes associated with aging, in *Aging and the Brain* (ed. C.M. Gaitz), 3rd edn, Plenum, New York.

Maletta, G.J., Pirozzolo, F.J., Thompson, G. and Mortimer, J.A. (1982) Organic mental disorders in a geriatric outpatient population. *Am. J. Psychiatry*, **139**, 521–3.

Mann, D.M.A., Yeates, P.O., Davies, J.S. and Hawkes, J. (1981)

Viruses, Parkinsonism and Alzheimer's disease. *J. Neurol. Neurosurg. Psychiatry*, **44**, 651.

Mant, A., Saunders, N.A., Eyland, A.E. *et al.* (1988) Sleep-related respiratory disturbance and dementia in elderly females. *J. Gerontol.: Med. Sci.*, **43**, 140–4.

Manton, K.G. (1986) Cause specific mortality patterns among the oldest old: Multiple cause of death trends 1968 to 1980. *J. Gerontol.*, **41**, 282–9.

Manuelidis, E.E., de Figueiredo, J.M., Kim, J.H. *et al.* (1988) Transmission studies from blood of Alzheimer disease patients and healthy relatives. *Proc. Natl Acad. Sci. USA*, **85**, 4898–901.

Marklund, S.L., Adolfsson, R., Gottfries, C.G. and Winblad, B. (1985) Superoxide dismutase isoenzymes in normal brains and in brains from patients with dementia of Alzheimer type. *J. Neurol. Sci.*, **67**, 319–25.

Marsden, C.D. and Harrison, M.J.G. (1972) Outcome of investigation of patients with presenile dementia. *Br. Med. J.*, **2**, 249–52.

Martin, D.C., Miller, J.K., Kapoor, W. *et al.* (1987a) A controlled study of survival with dementia. *Arch. Neurol.*, **44**, 1122–6.

Martin, E.M., Wilson, R.S., Penn, R.D. *et al.* (1987b) Cortical biopsy results in Alzheimer's disease: Correlation with cognitive deficits. *Neurology*, **37**, 1201–4.

Martin, R.L., Gerteis, G. and Gabrielli, W.F. (1988) A family-genetic study of dementia of Alzheimer type. *Arch. Gen. Psychiatry*, **45**, 894–900.

Marttila, R.J. and Rinne, U.K. (1988) Decrease of superoxide dismutase activity in the basal nucleus in Alzheimer's disease. *Acta Neurol. Scand.*, **77** (suppl. 116) 89.

Martyn, C.N. and Pippard, E.C. (1988) Usefulness of mortality data in determining the geography and time trends of dementia. *J. Epidemiol. Commun. Health*, **42**, 134–7.

Martyn, C.N., Barker, D.J.P., Osmond, C. *et al.* (1989) Geographical relation between Alzheimer's disease and aluminium in drinking water. *Lancet*, **i**, 59–62.

Masters, C.L., Gajdusek, D.C. and Gibbs, C.J. (1981) Creutzfeldt–Jakob disease virus isolation from the Gerstmann–Sträussler syndrome. *Brain*, **104**, 559–88.

Matsushita, M. and Ishii, T. (1979) Some problems on multi-infarct dementia. *Clin. Psychiatry*, **21**, 613–24 (in Japanese).

Matsuyama, H. and Nakamura, S. (1978) Senile changes in the brain in the Japanese: Incidence of Alzheimer's neurofibrillary change and senile plaques, in *Alzheimer's Disease: Senile Dementia and Related Disorders*. (eds R. Katzman, R.D. Terry and K.L. Bick), Raven Press, New York.

Maule, M.M., Milne, J.S. and Williamson, J. (1984) Mental illness and physical health in older people. *Age Ageing*, **13**, 239–56.

Mayer-Gross, W., Slater, E. and Roth, M. (1954) *Clinical Psychiatry*. Cassell, London.

Mayer-Gross, W., Slater, E. and Roth, M. (1960) *Clinical Psychiatry*, 2nd edn, Cassell, London.

Mayor, G.H., Keiser, J.A., Makdani, D. and Ku, P.K. (1977) Aluminum absorption and distribution: Effect of parathyroid hormone. *Science*, **197**, 1187–9.

Meaney, M.J., Aitken, D.H., van Berkel, C. *et al.* (1988) Effect of neonatal handling on age-related impairments associated with the hippocampus. *Science*, **239**, 766–8.

Medical Research Council (1987) *Report from the MRC Alzheimer's Disease Workshop*, Medical Research Council, Britain.

Meyer, J.S., Judd, B.W., Tawakina, T. *et al.* (1986) Improved cognition after control of risk factors for multi-infarct dementia. *J. Am. Med. Assoc.*, **256**, 2203–9.

Meyer, J.S., McClintic, K.L., Rogers, R.L. *et al.* (1988) Aetiological considerations and risk factors for multi-infarct dementia. *J. Neurol., Neurosurg. Psychiatry*, **51**, 1489–97.

Meyer, J.S., Rogers, R.L., McClintic, K. *et al.* (1989) Randomized clinical trial of daily aspirin therapy in multi-infarct dementia. *J. Am. Geriatr. Soc.*, **37**, 549–55.

Middleton, P.J., Petric, M., Kozak, M. *et al.* (1980) Herpes-simplex viral genome and senile and presenile dementias of Alzheimer and Pick. *Lancet*, **i**, 1038.

Mikkelsen, S. (1980) A cohort study of disability pension and death among painters with special regard to disabling presenile dementia as an occupational disease. *Scand. J. Soc. Med.*, **16**, 34–43.

Mikkelsen, S., Jørgensen, M., Browne, E. and Gyldensted, C. (1988) Mixed solvent exposure and organic brain damage: A study of painters. *Acta Neurol. Scand.*, **78** (suppl. 118), 1–143.

Miller, D.F., Hicks, S.P., D'Amato, C.J. and Landis, J.R. (1984) A descriptive study of neuritic plaques and neurofibrillary tangles in an autopsy population. *Am. J. Epidemiol.*, **120**, 331–41.

Mohs, R.C., Breitner, J.C.S., Silverman, J.M. and Davis, K.L. (1987) Alzheimer's disease. Morbid risk among first-degree relatives approximates 50% by 90 years of age. *Arch. Gen. Psychiatry*, **44**, 405–8.

Mölsä, P.K., Marttila, R.J. and Rinne, U.K. (1982) Epidemiology of dementia in a Finnish population. *Acta Neurol. Scand.*, **65**, 541–52.

Mölsä, P.K., Marttila, R.J. and Rinne, U.K. (1984) Mortality of patients with dementia. *Acta Neurol. Scand.*, **69** (suppl. 98), 230–1.

Mölsä, P., Paljärvi, L., Rinne, J.O. *et al* (1985) Validity of clinical diagnosis in dementia: A prospective clinicopathological study. *J. Neurol. Neurosurg. Psychiatry*, **48**, 1085–90.

Mölsä, P.K., Säkö, E., Paljärvi, L. (1988) Natural course in dementia. *Acta Neurol. Scand.*, **77** (suppl. 116), 89.

Morgan, K., Dallosso, H.M., Arie, T. *et al.* (1987) Mental health and psychological well-being among the old and the very old living at home. *Br. J. Psychiatry*, **150**, 801–7.

Morimatsu, M., Hirai, S., Muramatsu, A. and Yoshikawa, M. (1975) Senile degenerative brain lesions and dementia. *J. Am. Geriatr. Soc.*, **23**, 390–406.

Morris, J.C. (1989) Binswanger's disease or artifact: A clinical, neuro-imaging, and pathological study of periventricular white matter changes in Alzheimer's disease, in *Alzheimer's Disease* (eds R.J. Wurtman, S. Corkin, J.H. Growdon and E. Ritter-Walker), Proceedings of the Fifth Meeting of the International Study Group on the Pharmacology of Memory Disorders Associated with Aging, Zurich.

Morris, J.C., McKeel, D.W., Fulling, K. *et al.* (1988) Validation of clinical diagnostic criteria for Alzheimer's disease. *Ann. Neurol.*, **24**, 17–22.

Mortimer, J.A. (1988) Do psychosocial risk factors contribute to Alzheimer's disease? in *Etiology of Dementia of Alzheimer's Type* (eds A.S. Henderson and J.H. Henderson). John Wiley, Chichester.

Mortimer, J.A. (1989) Epidemiology of dementia: Cross-cultural comparisons, in *Alzheimer's Disease* (eds R.J. Wurtman, S. Corkin, J.H. Growdon and E. Ritter-Walker), Proceedings of the Fifth Meeting of the International Study Group on the Pharmacology of Memory Disorders Associated with Aging, Zurich.

Mortimer, J.A. and Schuman, L.M. (1981) *The Epidemiology of Dementia*, Oxford University Press, New York.

Mortimer, J.A., Schuman, L.M. and French, L.R. (1981) Epidemiology of dementing illness, in *The Epidemiology of Dementia* (eds J.A. Mortimer and L.M. Schuman), Oxford University Press, New York.

Mortimer, J.A., French, L.R., Hutton, J.T. and Schuman, L.M. (1985a) Head injury as a risk factor for Alzheimer's disease. *Neurology*, **35**, 264–7.

Mortimer, J.A., French, L.R., Schuman, L.M. and Hutton, J.T. (1985b) Head injuries in Alzheimer's disease and vascular dementia. *Neurology*, **35**, 1804.

Motohiro, S., Shimura, J., Ichimiya, A. *et al.* (1985) The prevalence study on age associated dementia in Fukuoka City. *Geriatr. Psychiatr.*, **2**, 919–27 (in Japanese).

Mowry, B.J. and Burvill, P.W. (1988) A study of mild dementia in the community using a wide range of diagnostic criteria. *Br. J. Psychiatry*, **153**, 328–34.

Muckle, T.J. and Roy, J.R. (1985) High-density lipoprotein cholesterol in differential diagnosis of senile dementia. *Lancet*, **i**, 1191–2.

Müller, H.F. and Schwartz, G. (1978) Electroencephalograms and autopsy findings in geropsychiatry. *J. Gerontol.*, **33**, 504–13.

Murray, R.M., Greene, J.G. and Adams, J.H. (1971) Analgesic abuse and dementia. *Lancet*, **ii**, 242–5.

Myers, J.K., Weissman, M.M., Tischler, G.L. *et al.* (1984) Six-month prevalence of psychiatric disorders in three communities. *Arch. Gen. Psychiatry*, **41**, 959–67.

National Institutes of Health (1987) *Differential diagnosis of dementing diseases*, US Department of Health and Human Services, Bethesda.

Nee, L.E., Eldridge, R., Sunderland, T. *et al.* (1987) Dementia of the Alzheimer type: Clinical and family study of 22 twin pairs. *Neurology*, **37**, 359–63.

Newman, S.C. and Bland, R.C. (1987) Canadian trends in mortality from mental disorders, 1965–1983. *Acta Psychiatr. Scand.*, **76**, 1–7.

Nielsen, B., Gunner-Svensson, F., Friborg, S. and Olsen, J. (1982) Praevalens af svaer demens blandt aeldrei Odense kommune, 1972. *Fagligt og Socialt, 144/146*, 3455–7.

Nielsen, J. (1962) Geronto-psychiatric period-prevalence investigation in a geographically delimited population. *Acta Psychiatr. Scand.*, **38**, 307–30.

Nielsen, J.A., Biørn-Henriksen, T. and Bork, B.R. (1981) Incidence and disease expectancy for senile and arteriosclerotic dementia in a geographically delimited Danish rural population, in *Epidemiology and Prevention of Mental Illness in Old Age* (eds G. Magnussen, J. Nielsen and J. Buch), Nordisk Samråd for Eldreaktivitet, Hellerup.

Nilsson, L.V. (1984) Incidence of severe dementia in an urban sample followed from 70 to 79 years of age. *Acta Psychiatr. Scand.*, **70**, 478–86.

Nilsson, L.V. and Persson, G. (1984) Prevalence of mental disorders in an urban sample examined at 70, 75 and 79 years of age. *Acta Psychiatr. Scand.*, **69**, 519–27.

Nishihara, Y. and Ishii, N. (1986) Pathological study of demented old people in Japan. *Kyushu Neuropsychiatry*, **31**, 41–5.

O'Connor, D.W., Pollitt, P.A., Hyde, J.B. *et al.* (1988) Do general practitioners miss dementia in elderly patients? *Br. Med. J.*, **297**, 1107–10.

O'Connor, D.W., Pollitt, P.A., Hyde, J.B. *et al.* (1989a) The reliability and validity of the Mini-Mental State in a British community survey. *J. Psychiatr. Res.*, **23**, 87–96.

O'Connor, D.W., Pollitt, P.A., Treasure, F.P. *et al.* (1989b). The influence of education, social class and sex on Mini-Mental State scores. *Psychol. Med.*, **19**, 771–6.

O'Connor, D.W., Pollitt, P.A., Hyde, J.B. *et al.* (1989c) The prevalence of dementia as measured by the Cambridge Mental Disorders of the Elderly Examination. *Acta Psychiatr. Scand.*, **79**, 190–8.

Ojeda, V., Mastaglia, F.L. and Kakulas, B.A. (1986) Causes of organic dementia: A necropsy survey of 60 cases. *Med. J. Aust.*, **145**, 69–71.

Oliver, C. and Holland, A.J. (1986) Down's syndrome and Alzheimer's disease: a review. *Psychol. Med.*, **16**, 307–22.

Omura, T., Hisamatsu, S., Takizawa, Y. *et al.* (1987) Geographical distribution of cerebrovascular disease mortality and food intakes in Japan. *Soc Sci. Med.*, **24**, 401–7.

Park, J-H. and Ha, J.C. (1988) Cognitive impairment among the elderly in a Korean rural community. *Acta Psychiatr. Scand.*, **77**, 52–7.

Parsons, P.L. (1965) Mental health in Swansea's old folk. *Br. J. Prev. Soc. Med.*, **19**, 43–7.

Pasamanick, B., Roberts, D.W., Lemkau, P.V. and Krueger, D.E. (1957) A survey of mental disease in an urban population. I. Prevalence by age, sex and severity of impairment. *Am. J. Pub. Health*, **47**, 923–9.

Pattie, A.H. (1981) A survey version of the Clifton Assessment Procedures for the Elderly (CAPE). *Br. J. Clin. Psychol.*, **20**, 173–8.

Pattie, A.H. and Gilleard, C.J. (1975) A brief psychogeriatric schedule. Validation against psychiatric diagnosis and discharge from hospital. *Br. J. Psychiatry*, **127**, 489–93.

Pattie, A.H. and Gilleard, C.J. (1976) The Clifton Assessment Schedule – further validation of a psychogeriatric assessment schedule. *Br. J. Psychiatry*, **129**, 68–72.

Pattie, A.H. and Gilleard, C.J. (1978) The two-year predictive validity of the Clifton Assessment Schedule and the shortened Stockton Geriatric Rating Scale. *Br. J. Psychiatry*, **133**, 457–60.

Pattie, A.H. and Gilleard, C.J. (1979) *Clifton Assessment Procedures for the Elderly (CAPE) Specimen Set*, Hodder and Stoughton, Kent.

Pearce, F. (1985) Acid rain may cause senile dementia. *New Sci.*, **106**, 7.

Peck, A., Wolloch, L. and Rodstein, M. (1978) Mortality of the aged with chronic brain syndrome: Further observations in a five-year study. *J. Am. Geriatr. Soc.*, **26**, 170–6.

Pentz, C.A., Elias, M.F., Wood, W.G. *et al.* (1979) Relationship of age and hypertension to neuropsychological test performance. *Exp. Aging Res.*, **5**, 351–72.

Peress, N.S., Kane, W.C. and Aronson, S.M. (1978) Central nervous system findings in a tenth decade autopsy population. *Prog. Brain Res.*, **40**, 473–83.

Perl, D.P. and Good, P.F. (1987) Uptake of aluminium into central nervous system along nasal-olfactory pathways. *Lancet*, **i**, 1028.

Peto, R., Gray, R., Collins, R. *et al.* (1988) Randomised trial of prophylactic daily aspirin in British male doctors. *Br. Med. J.*, **296**, 313–16.

Pfeiffer, E. (1975) A short portable mental status questionnaire for the assessment of organic brain deficit in elderly patients. *J. Am. Geriatr. Soc.*, **23**, 433–41.

Pickle, L.W., Brown, L.M. and Blot, W.J. (1983) Information available from surrogate respondents in case-control interview studies. *Am J. Epidemiol.*, **118**, 99–108.

Pinessi, L., Rainero, I., Angelini, G. *et al.* (1983) I fattori di rischio nelle sindromi demenziali primarie. *Minerva Psichiatrica*, **24**, 87–91.

Pinessi, L., Rainero, I., Asteggiano, G. *et al.* (1984) Primary dementias: Epidemiological and sociomedical aspects. *Ital. J. Neurol. Sci.*, **5**, 51–5.

Podlisny, M.B., Lee, G. and Selkoe, D.J. (1987) Gene dosage of the amyloid β precursor protein in Alzheimer's disease. *Science*, **238**, 669–71.

Podrabinek, O., Roudier, M., Lamour, Y. and de Grouchy, J. (1988) Dermatoglyphic patterns in senile dementia of Alzheimer's type. *Ann. Génét.*, **31**, 91–6.

Preston, G.A.N. (1986) Dementia in elderly adults: Prevalence and institutionalization. *J. Gerontol.*, **41**, 261–7.

Primrose, E.J.R. (1962) *Psychological Illness: A Community Study.* Charles C. Thomas, Springfield, Illinois.

Prusiner, S.B. (1982) Novel proteinaceous infectious particles cause scrapie. *Science*, **216**, 136–44.

Prusiner, S.B. (1984) Some speculations about prions, amyloid and Alzheimer's disease. *New Engl. J. Med.*, **310**, 661–3.

Rabins, P.V. (1981) The prevalence of reversible dementia in a psychiatric hopsital. *Hospital and Community Psychiatry*, **32**, 490–2.

Reding, M.J., Haycox, J., Wigforss, K. *et al.* (1984) Follow-up of patients referred to a dementia service. *J. Am. Geriatr. Soc.*, **32**, 265–8.

Reding, M.J., Haycox, J. and Blass, J.P. (1985) Depression in patients referred to a dementia clinic: A three-year prospective study. *Archives of Neurology*, **42**, 894–6.

Reimann, H. and Häfner, H. (1972) Psychische Erkrankungen alter Menschen in Mannheim. *Soc. Psychiatr*, **7**, 53–69.

Reisberg, B., Ferris, S.H., de Leon, M.J. and Crook, T. (1982) The global deterioration scale for assessment of primary degenerative dementia. *Am. J. Psychiatry*, **139**, 1136–9.

Reynolds, C.F., Kupfer, D.J., Taska, L.S. *et al.* (1985) Sleep apnea in Alzheimer's dementia: Correlation with mental deterioration. *J. Clin. Psychiatry*, **46**, 257–61.

Reynolds, C.R. (1982) Methods for detecting construct and predictive bias, in *Handbook of Methods for Detecting Test Bias* (ed. R.A. Berk), Johns Hopkins University Press, Baltimore and London.

Ridley, R.M., Baker, H.F. and Crow, T.J. (1986) Transmissible and non-transmissible neurodegenerative disease: similarities in age of onset and genetics in relation to aetiology. *Psychol. Med.*, **16**, 199–207.

Rimm, A.A. (1986) Re: 'A case-control study of dementia of the Alzheimer type'. *Am. J. Edpidemiol.*, **123**, 753.

Robakis, N.K., Wisniewski, H.M., Jenkins, E.C. *et al.* (1987) Chromosome 21q21 sublocalisation of gene encoding beta-amyloid peptide in cerebral vessels and neuritic (senile) plaques of people with Alzheimer disease and Down syndrome. *Lancet*, **i**, 384–5.

Roberts, E. (1986) Alzheimer's disease may begin in the nose and may be caused by aluminosilicates. *Neurobiol. Aging*, **7**, 561–7.

Roberts, G.W., Lofthouse, R., Brown R. *et al.* (1986) Prion-protein immunoreactivity in human transmissible dementias. *New Engl. J. Med.*, **315**, 1231–3.

Robertson, D., Rockwood, K. and Stolee, P. (1984) *Prevalence of Dementia in the Elderly of Saskatchewan*, Unpublished manuscript, Division of Geriatric Medicine, University of Saskatchewan.

Rocca, W.A. and Amaducci, L. (1984) Proiezioni demografiche per la popolazione anziana trail 1980 ed il 2000: possibili conceguenze per la prevalenza della demenza senile. In *Atti dela '85 congresso della societa Italiana di medicina interna*, (Vol. I), Roma.

Rocca, W.A., Fratiglioni, L., Bracco, L. *et al.* (1986) The use of surrogate respondents to obtain questionnaire data in case-control studies of neurologic diseases. *J. Chronic Dis.*, **39**, 907–12.

Roman, G.C. (1987) Senile dementia of the Binswanger type: A vascular form of dementia in the elderly. *J. Am. Med. Assoc.*, **258**, 1782–8.

Rorsman, B., Hagnell, O. and Lanke, J. (1985a) Prevalence of age psychosis and mortality among age psychotics in the Lundby study. *Neuropsychobiology*, **13**, 167–72.

Rorsman, B., Hagnell, O. and Lanke, J. (1985b) Mortality and age psychosis in the Lundby study: Death risk of senile and multi-infarct dementia *Neuropsychobiology*, **14**, 13–16.

Rorsman, B., Hagnell, O, and Lanke, J. (1986) Prevalence and incidence of senile and multi-infarct dementia in the Lundby study: A comparison between the time periods 1947–1957 and 1957–1972. *Neuropsychobiology*, **15**, 122–9.

Rosen, W.G., Terry, R.D., Fuld, P.A. *et al.* (1980) Pathological verification of ischemic score in the differentiation of dementia. *Ann. Neurol.*, **7**, 466–8.

Roses, A.D., Pericak-Vance, M.A., Clark, C.M. *et al.* (1989) Linkage studies in late onset familial Alzheimer's disease, in *Alzheimer's Disease* (eds R.J. Wurtman, S. Corkin, J.H Growdon and E. Ritter-Walker), Proceedings of the Fifth Meeting of the International Study Group on the Pharmacology of Memory Disorders Associated with Aging, Zurich.

Roth, M. (1955) The natural history of mental disorder in old age. *J. Ment. Sci.*, **101**, 281–301.

Roth, M. (1981) The diagnosis of dementia in late and middle life, in *The Epidemiology of Dementia* (eds J.A. Mortimer and L.M. Schuman), Oxford University Press, New York.

Roth, M. (1986) The association of clinical and neurological findings and its bearing on the classification and aetiology of Alzheimer's disease *Br. Med. Bull.*, **42**, 42–50.

Roth, M., Tym, E., Mountjoy, C.Q. *et al.* (1986) CAMDEX. A standardised instrument for the diagnosis of mental disorder in the elderly with special reference for the early detection of dementia. *Br J. Psychiatry*, **149**, 698–709.

Roth, M., Huppert, F.A. Tym, E. and Mountjoy, C.Q. (1988) *CAMDEX: the Cambridge Examination for Mental Disorders of the Elderly*, Cambridge University Press, Cambridge.

Rowe, I.F., Ridler, M.A.C. and Gibberd, F.B. (1989) Presenile dementia associated with mosaic trisomy 21 in a patient with a Down syndrome child. *Lancet*, **ii**, 229.

Rudelli, R., Strom, J.O., Welch, P.T. and Ambler, M.W. (1982) Post-traumatic premature Alzheimer's disease: Neuropathologic findings and pathogenetic consideration. *Arch. Neurol*, **39**, 570–5.

Saugstad, L.F. and Ødegård, Ø. (1979) Mortality in psychiatric hospitals in Norway 1950–74. *Acta Psychiatr. Scand.*, 59, 431–47.

Savory, J., Nicholson, J.R. and Wills, M.R. (1987) Is aluminium leaching enhanced by fluoride? *Nature*, **327**, 107–8.

Sayetta, R.B. (1986) Rates of senile dementia – Alzheimer's type in the Baltimore longitudinal study. *J. Chronic Dis.*, **39**, 271–86.

Schaie, K.W. (1984) Midlife influences upon intellectual functioning in old age. *Int. J. Behav. Dev.*, **7**, 463–78.

Schaie, K.W. and Willis, S.L. (1986) Can decline in adult intellectual functioning be reversed? *Dev. Psychol.*, **22**, 223–32.

Scheinberg, P. (1988) Dementia due to vascular disease – a multifactorial disorder. *Stroke*, **19**, 1291–9.

Schellenberg, G.D., Bird, T.D., Wijsman, E.M. *et al.* (1988) Absence of linkage of chromsome 21q21 markers to familial Alzheimer's disease. *Science*, **241**, 1507–9.

Scherr, P.A., Albert M.S., Funkenstein, H.H. *et al.* (1988) Correlates of cognitive function in an elderly community population. *Am. J. Epidemiol.*, **128**, 1084–101.

Schlesselman, J.L. (1982) *Case-control studies: Design, conduct, analysis*, Oxford University Press, New York.

Schoenberg, B.S., Okazaki, H. and Kokmen, E. (1981) Reduced survival in patients with dementia: A population study. *Trans. Am. Neurol. Assoc.*, **106**, 306–8.

Schoenberg, B.S., Anderson, D.W. and Haerer, A.F. (1985) Severe dementia: Prevalence and clinical features in a biracial US population. *Arch. Neurol.*, **42**, 740–3.

Schoenberg, B.S., Kokmen, E. and Okazaki, H. (1987) Alzheimer's disease and other dementing illnesses in a defined United States population: Incidence rates and clinical features. *Ann. Neurol.*, **22**, 724–9.

Schoenberg, B.S., Rocca, W.A., Fratiglioni, L. *et al.* (1988) Late maternal age as a risk factor for sporadic and familial Alzheimer's disease (AD). *Neurology,* **38** (suppl. 1), 311.

Schultz, N.R., Dineen, J.T., Elias, M.F. *et al.* (1979) WAIS performance for different age groups of hypertensive and control subjects during the administration of a diuretic. *J. Gerontol.,* **34**, 246–53.

Selnes, O.A., Carson, K., Rovner, B. and Gordon, B. (1988) Language dysfunction in early- and late-onset possible Alzheimer's disease. *Neurology,* **38**, 1053–6.

Seltzer, B. and Sherwin, I. (1983) A comparison of clinical features in early- and late-onset primary degenerative dementia: One entity or two? *Arch. Neurol.,* **40**, 143–6.

Seltzer, B. and Sherwin, I. (1986) Fingerprint pattern differences in early- and late-onset primary degenerative dementia. *Arch. Neurol.,* **43**, 665–8.

Seltzer, B., Burres, M.J.K. and Sherwin, I. (1984) Left-handedness in early- and late-onset dementia. *Neurology,* **34**, 367–9.

Sequiera, L.W., Jennings, L.C., Carrasco, L.H. *et al.* (1979) Detection of herpes simplex virus genome in brain tissue. *Lancet,* **ii**, 609–12.

Shah, K.V., Banks, G.D. and Merskey, H. (1969) Survival in athero-sclerotic and senile dementia. *Br. J. Psychiatry,* **115**, 1283–6.

Shalat, S.L., Seltzer, B., Pidcock, C. and Baker, E.L. (1987) Risk factors for Alzheimer's disease: A case-control study. *Neurology,* **37**, 1630–3.

Shalat, S.L., Seltzer, B. and Baker, E.L. (1988) Occupational risk factors and Alzheimer's disease: A case-control study. *J. Occup. Med.,* **30**, 934–6.

Shefer, V.F. (1987) Hypo- and hyperdiagnosis of senile dementia and Alzheimer's disease in psychiatric practice. *Zh. Nevropatol. Psikhiatr.,* **87**, 987–92 (in Russian).

Sheldon, J.H. (1948) *The Social Medicine of Old Age,* Oxford University Press, London.

Shibayama, H., Kasahara, Y., Kobayashi, H. *et al.* (1986) Prevalence of dementia in a Japanese elderly population. *Acta Psychiatr. Scand.,* **74**, 144–51.

Shore, D. and Wyatt, R.J. (1983) Aluminium and Alzheimer's disease. *J. Nerv. Ment. Dis.,* **171**, 553–8.

Silverstein, A.B., Herbs, D., Nasuta, R. and White, J.F. (1986) Effects of age on the adaptive behavior of institutionalized individuals with Down syndrome. *Am. J. Ment. Defic.,* **90**, 659–62.

Sinet, P.M. (1982) Metabolism of oxygen derivatives in Down's syndrome. *Ann. N. Y. Acad. Sci.,* **396**, 83–94.

Sjögren, T., Sjögren, H. and Lindgren, A.G.H. (1952) Morbus Alzheimer and morbus Pick: A genetic, clinical and patho-anatomical study. *Acta Psychiatr. Neurol. Scand.,* (suppl. 82), 1–109.

Skullerud, K. (1985) Variations in the size of the human brain: Influence of age, sex, body length, body mass index, alcoholism, Alzheimer changes, and cerebral atherosclerosis. *Acta Neurol. Scand.*, **71** (suppl. 102), 1–93.

Small, G.W. (1985) Revised ischemic score for diagnosing multi-infarct dementia. *J. Clin. Psychiatry*, **46**, 514–17.

Small, G.W., Matsuyama, S.S., Komanduri, R. *et al.* (1985) Thyroid disease in patients with dementia of the Alzheimer type. *J. Am. Geriatr. Soc.*, **33**, 538–9.

Smallwood, R.G., Vitiello, M.V., Giblin, E.C. and Prinz, P.N. (1983) Sleep apnea: Relationship to age, sex, and Alzheimer's dementia. *Sleep*, **6**, 16–22.

Smirne, S., Franceschi, M., Bareggi, S.R. *et al.* (1981) Sleep apneas in Alzheimer's disease, in *Sleep 1980, 5th European Congress on Sleep Research, Amsterdam*, Karger, Basel.

Smith, J.S. and Kiloh, L.G. (1981) The investigation of dementia: Results in 200 consecutive admissions. *Lancet*, i, 824–7.

Soininen, H. and Heinonen, O.P. (1982) Clinical and etiological aspects of senile dementia. *Eur. Neurol.*, **21**, 401–10.

Sourander, P. and Sjögren, H. (1970) The concept of Alzheimer's disease and its clinical implications, in *Alzheimer's Disease and Related Conditions* (eds G.E.W. Wolstenholme and M. O'Connor), Churchill Livingstone, London.

Spencer, P.S., Nunn, P.B., Hugon, J. *et al.* (1987) Guam amyotrophic lateral sclerosis–parkinsonism–dementia linked to a plant excitant neurotoxin. *Science*, **237**, 517–22.

Stam, F.C., Wigboldus, J.M. and Smeulders, A.W.M. (1986) Age incidence of senile brain amyloidosis. *Pathol. Res. Pract.*, **181**, 558–62.

St Clair, D. and Whalley, L.J. (1983) Hypertension, multi-infarct dementia and Alzheimer's disease. *Br. J. Psychiatry*, **143**, 274–6.

Steering Committee of the Physicians' Health Study Research Group (1989) Final report on the aspirin component of the ongoing physicians' health study. *New Engl. J. Med.*, **321**, 129–35.

Sternberg, E. and Gawrilowa, S. (1978) Über klinisch-epidemiologische Untersuchungen in der sowjetischen Alterspsychiatrie. *Nervenarzt*, **49**, 347–53.

St George-Hyslop, P.H., Tanzi, R.E., Polinsky, R.J., Neve, R.L. *et al.* (1987a) Absence of duplication of chromosome 21 genes in familial and sporadic Alzheimer's disease. *Science*, **238**, 664–6.

St George-Hyslop, P.H., Tanzi, R.E., Polinsky, R.J. *et al.* (1987b) The genetic defect causing familial Alzheimer's disease maps on chromosome 21. *Science*, **235**, 885–90.

Storandt, M., Aufdembrinke, B., Bäckman, L. *et al.* (1988) Relationship of normal aging and dementing diseases in later life, in *Etiology of Dementia of Alzheimer's Type* (eds A.S. Henderson and J.H. Henderson), John Wiley, Chichester.

Struwe, F. (1929) Histopathologische Untersuchungen über Entstehung und Wesen der senilen plaques. Zeitschrift für die gesamte. *Neurol. Psychiatr.*, **122**, 291.

Sulkava, R. and Erkinjuntti, T. (1987) Vascular dementia due to cardiac arrhythmias and systemic hypotension. *Acta Neurol. Scand.*, **76**, 123–8.

Sulkava, R., Haltia, M., Paetau, A. *et al.* (1983) Accuracy of clinical diagnosis in primary degenerative dementia: Correlation with neuropathological findings. *J. Neurol., Neurosurg. Psychiatry*, **46**, 9–13.

Sulkava, R., Wikström, J., Aromaa, A. *et al.* (1985a) Prevalence of severe dementia in Finland. *Neurology*, **35**, 1025–9.

Sulkava, R., Erkinjuntti, T. and Palo, J. (1985b) Head injuries in Alzheimer's disease and vascular dementia. *Neurology*, **35**, 1084.

Sulkava, R., Heliövaara, M., Palo, J. *et al.* (1988) Regional differences in the prevalence of Alzheimer's disease. *Proceedings of the International Symposium on Alzheimer's Disease*, Department of Neurology, University of Kuopio, Finland.

Talamo, B.R., Rudel, R.A., Kosik, K.S. *et al.* (1989) Pathological changes in olfactory neurons in patients with Alzheimer's disease. *Nature*, **337**, 736–9.

Tanzi, R.E., Gusella, J.F., Watkins, P.C. *et al.* (1987a) Amyloid β protein gene: cDNA, mRNA distribution, and genetic linkage near the Alzheimer locus. *Science*, **235**, 880–4.

Tanzi, R.E., St George-Hyslop, P.H., Haines, J.L. *et al.* (1987b) The genetic defect in familial Alzheimer's disease is not tightly linked to the amyloid β-protein gene. *Nature*, **329**, 156–7.

Taylor, E. and Devakumar, M. (1989) Aluminium and Alzheimer's disease. *Lancet*, **i**, 267.

Teasdale, T.W. and Owen, D.R. (1987) National secular trends in intelligence and education: a twenty-year cross-sectional study. *Nature*, **325**, 119–21.

Tennakone, K. and Wickramanayake, S. (1987a) Aluminium leaching from cooking utensils. *Nature*, **325**, 202.

Tennakone, K. and Wickramanayake, S. (1987b) Aluminium and cooking. *Nature*, **329**, 398.

Terry, R.D. and Wisniewski, H.M. (1970) The ultrastructure of the neurofibrillary tangle and the senile plaque, in *Alzheimer's Disease and Related Conditions*, (eds G.E.W. Wolstenholme and M. O'Connor), Churchill Livingstone, London.

Thal, L.J., Grundman, M. and Klauber, M.R. (1988) Dementia: Characteristics of a referral population and factors associated with progression. *Neurology*, **38**, 1083–90.

Thase, M.E., Tigner, R., Smeltzer, D.J. and Liss, L. (1984) Age-related neuropsychological deficits in Down's syndrome. *Biol. Psychiatry*, **19**, 571–85.

Thompson, E.G. and Eastwood, M.R. (1981) Survivorship and senile dementia. *Age Ageing*, **10**, 29–32.

Thygesen, P., Hermann, K. and Willanger, R. (1970) Concentration camp survivors in Denmark. Persecution, disease, disability, compensation. A 23-year follow-up. A survey of the long-term effects of severe environmental stress. *Dan. Med. Bull.*, **17**, 65–108.

Tierney, M.C., Fisher, R.H., Lewis, A.J. *et al.* (1988) The NINCDS–ADRDA Work Group criteria for the clinical diagnosis of probable Alzheimer's disease: A clinicopathologic study of 57 cases. *Neurology*, **38**, 359–64.

Todorov, A.B., Go, R.C.P., Constantinidis, J. and Elston, R.C. (1975) Specificity of the clinical diagnosis of dementia. *J. Neurol. Sci.*, **26**, 81–98.

Tomlinson, B.E. and Kitchener, D. (1972) Granulovacuolar degeneration of hippocampal pyramidal cells. *J. Pathol.*, **106**, 165–85.

Tomlinson, B. E., Blessed, G. and Roth, M. (1970) Observations on the brains of demented old people. *J. Neurol. Sci.*, **11**, 205–42.

Tomonaga, M. (1979) Studies on the morphological background of dementia in old age – A clinicopathological investigation on the cases with abundant senile plaques. *Jpn J. Geriatr.*, **16**, 1–6 (in Japanese).

Trapp, G.A. and Cannon, J.B. (1981) Aluminum pots as a source of dietary aluminium. *New Engl. J. Med.*, **304**, 172.

Treves, T., Korczyn, A.D., Zilber, N. *et al.* (1986) Presenile dementia in Israel. *Arch. Neurol.*, **43**, 26–9.

Ueda, K., Omae, T., Hirota, Y. *et al.* (1981) Decreasing trend in incidence and mortality from stroke in Hisayama residents, Japan. *Stroke*, **12**, 154–60.

Ulrich, J. (1985) Alzheimer changes in nondemented patients younger than sixty-five: Possible early stages of Alzheimer's disease and senile dementia of Alzheimer type. *Ann. Neurol.*, **17**, 273–7.

Urakami, K., Adachi, Y. and Takahashi, K. (1988) A community-based study of parental age in Alzheimer-type dementia in western Japan. *Arch. Neurol.*, **45**, 375.

Van Broeckhoven, C., Genthe, A.M., Vandenberghe, A. *et al.* (1987) Failure of familial Alzheimer's disease to segregate with the A4-amyloid gene in several European families. *Nature*, **329**, 153–5.

Van Duijn, C.M., Tanja, T.A., Haaxma, R. *et al.* (1989) *Head trauma and sporadic Alzheimer's disease.* Unpublished manuscript, Erasmus University Medical School, Rotterdam.

Varsamis, J., Zuchowski, T. and Maini, K.K. (1972) Survival rates and causes of death in geriatric psychiatric patients. *Can. Psychiatr. Assoc. J.*, **17**, 17–22.

Victoratos, G.C., Lenman, J.A.R. and Herzberg, L. (1977) Neurological investigation of dementia. *Br. J. Psychiatry*, **130**, 131–3.

Vitaliano, P.P., Peck, A., Johnson, D.A. *et al.* (1981) Dementia and other competing risks for mortality in the institutionalized aged. *J. Am. Geriatr. Soc.*, **29**, 513–19.

Vogt, J. (1986) *Vannkvalitet og helse: Analyse av en mulig sammenheng mellom aluminium i drikkevann og aldersdemens*, Statistisk Sentralbyrå, Oslo.

Wade, J.P.H. and Hachinski, V.C. (1987) Multi-infarct dementia, in *Dementia* (ed. B. Pitt), Churchill Livingstone, Edinburgh.

Wade, J.P.H., Mirsen, T.R., Hachinski, V.C. *et al.* (1987) The clinical diagnosis of Alzheimer's disease. *Arch. Neurol.*, **44**, 24–9.

Walker, A.M., Martin-Moreno, J.M. and Artalejo, F.R. (1988) Odd man out: A graphical approach to meta-analysis. *Am. J. Pub. Health*, **78**, 961–6.

Wallace, R.B., Lemke, J.H., Morris, M.C. *et al.* (1985) Relationship of free-recall memory to hypertension in the elderly. The Iowa 65+ rural health study. *J. Chronic Dis.*, **38**, 475–81.

Weinreb, H.J. (1985) Fingerprint patterns in Alzheimer's disease. *Arch. Neurol.*, **42**, 50–4.

Weinreb, H.J. (1986) Dermatoglyphic patterns in Alzheimer's disease. *J. Neurogenet.*, **3**, 233–46.

Weissman, M.M., Myers, J.K., Tischler, G.L. *et al.* (1985) Psychiatric disorders (DSM-III) and cognitive impairment in the elderly in a U.S. urban community. *Acta Psychiatr. Scand.*, **71**, 366–79.

Weyerer, S. (1983) Mental disorders among the elderly. True prevalence and use of medical services. *Arch. Gerontol. Geriatr.*, **2**, 11–22.

Whalley, L.J., Urbaniak, S.J., Darg, C. *et al.* (1980) Histocompatibility antigens and antibodies to viral and other antigens in Alzheimer pre-senile dementia. *Acta Psychiatr. Scand.*, **61**, 1–7.

Whalley, L.J., Darothers, A.D., Collyer, S. *et al.* (1982) A study of familial factors in Alzheimer's disease. *Br. J. Psychiatry*, **140**, 249–56.

White, J.A., McGue, M. and Heston, L.L. (1986) Fertility and parental age in Alzheimer disease. *J. Gerontol.*, **41**, 40–3.

Wilcock, G.K. and Esiri, M.M. (1982) Plaques, tangles and dementia: A quantitative study. *J. Neurol. Sci.*, **56**, 343–56.

Wilkie, F. and Eisdorfer, C. (1971) Intelligence and blood pressure in the aged. *Science*, **172**, 959–62.

Williamson, J., Stockoe, I.H., Gray, S. *et al.* (1964) Old people at home: their unreported needs. *Lancet*, **i**, 1117–20.

Wing. J.K. and Hailey, A.M. (1972) *Evaluating a Community Psychiatric Service*, Oxford University Press, London.

Wisniewski, H.M. and Rabe, A. (1986) Discrepancy between Alzheimer-type neuropathology and dementia in persons with Down's syndrome. *Ann. N. Y. Acad. Sci.*, **477**, 247–60.

Wisniewski, H.M., Merz, G.S. and Carp, R.I. (1984) Senile dementia of the Alzheimer type: Possibility of infectious etiology in genetically susceptible individuals. *Acta Neurol. Scand.*, **69** (suppl. 99), 91–7.

Wisniewski, K.E., Wisniewski, H.M. and Wen, G.Y. (1985) Occurrence of neuropathological changes and dementia of Alzheimer's disease in Down's syndrome. *Ann. Neurol.*, **17**, 278–82.

Wood, D.J., Cooper, C., Stevens, J. and Edwardson, J. (1988) Bone mass and dementia in hip fracture patients from areas with different aluminium concentrations in water supplies. *Age Ageing*, **17**, 415–19.

World Health Organization (1974) *Glossary of Mental Disorders and Guide to their Classification*, World Health Organization, Geneva.

World Health Organization (1978) *Mental Disorders: Glossary and Guide to their Classification in Accordance with the Ninth Revision of the International Classification of Diseases*, World Health Organization, Geneva.

Wright, A.F. and Whalley, L.J. (1984) Genetics, ageing and dementia. *Br. J. Psychiatry*, **145**, 20–38.

Yates, C.M., Simpson, J., Maloney, A.F.J. *et al.* (1980) Alzheimer-like cholinergic deficiency in Down's Syndrome. *Lancet*, **ii**, 979.

Yatham, L.N., McHale, P.A. and Kinsella, A. (1988) Down's syndrome and its association with Alzheimer's disease. *Acta Psychiatr. Scand.*, **77**, 38–41.

Yu, E.S.H., Liu, W.T., Levy, P. *et al.* (1989) Cognitive impairment among elderly adults in Shanghai, China. *J. Gerontol.: Soc. Sci.*, **44**, S97–106.

Zanetti, O., Rozzini, R., Bianchetti, A. and Trabucchi, M. (1985) HDL-cholesterol in dementia. *Lancet*, **ii**, 43.

Zhao, Y.Z. (1986) The epidemiological study of psychoses of different kinds, drug and alcohol dependence and personality disorders in 12 different regions of China. *Chin. J. Neurol. Psychiatr.*, **19**, 70–1 (in Chinese).

Zigman, W.B., Schupf, N., Lubin, R.A. and Silverman, W.P. (1987) Premature regression of adults with Down's syndrome. *Am. J. Ment. Defic.*, **92**, 161–8.

Zubenko, G.S., Wusylko, M., Cohen, B.M. *et al.* (1987) Family study of platelet membrane fluidity in Alzheimer's disease. *Science*, **238**, 539–42.

Zubenko, G.S., Huff, F.J., Beyer, J. *et al.* (1988) Familial risk of dementia associated with a biologic subtype of Alzheimer's disease. *Arch. Gen. Psychiatry*, **45**, 889–93.

Author Index

Subject Index